Daily Weight Loss Planner

Your key tool to healthy weight loss!

90 day planner
Created by: Rochelle Young, Registered Dietitian
Women's Edition

This Planner Belongs to:

Name: _______________________________

Telephone: _______________________________

Email: _______________________________

Everyday Tips for Healthy Weight Loss

Tip #1: Count your calories and fat!

Calories and fat contribute directly to weight gain. The less you eat of it, the more you will lose. The more calories and fat you eat, the more you will gain!

Tip #2: Know the amount of calories you need to limit yourself to daily to promote weight loss

Caloric needs for weight loss are determined by current weight. Below is a standard chart, however it is best to seek guidance from a Registered Dietitian for a more accurate calculation.

Current weight	Daily calorie goal	Daily fat goal
120-174#	1,200	33
175-219#	1,500	42
220-249#	1,800	50
250+	2000	55

Tip #3: Read your labels

When reading labels, your top priorities should be calorie and fat content. Be sure to check the serving size and do the necessary math!

Tip #4: Cook your meals and prep for the week

When we eat out, it's easier to encounter high calorie and fat foods. Save your calories and money by cooking and prepping your meals at home.

Tip #5: Get physical activity at least 30 minutes per day; five days per week

We all know exercising is a key element to weight loss. Try to burn at least half the calories or more you consume each day. Excerise also reduces risk for several chronic disases such as diabetes, hypertension and heart disease.

Plate Planner

Use food examples interchangeably, or choose your own similar food from the same food group!

Make half of your plate veggies!

- Green Salads
- Broccoli
-Cauliflower
- Green Beans
- Okra
- Mustard Greens
- Asparagus
- Zucchini
- Squash
- Mushrooms
- Carrots

1/4 protien

- Baked Chicken
- Baked fish (any type)
- Ground turkey
-Salisbury Steak
- Beef tips
- Turkey sausage

1/4 starch

- Brown rice
- Pasta noodles
-Mashed potatoes
- 1 small baked potato
- Corn
- Sweet peas

Reading Food Labels

Nutrition Facts

Serving Size 1 cup (228g)
Servings Per Container 2

Amount Per Serving

Calories 250	Calories from Fat 110
	% Daily Value*
Total Fat 12g	**18%**
Saturated Fat 3g	**15%**
Trans Fat 3g	
Cholesterol 30mg	**10%**
Sodium 470mg	**20%**
Potassium 700mg	**20%**
Total Carbohydrate 31g	**10%**
Dietary Fiber 0g	0%
Sugars 5g	
Protein 5g	
Vitamin A	4%
Vitamin C	2%
Calcium	20%
Iron	4%

* Percent Daily Values are based on a 2,000 calorie diet. Your Daily Values may be higher or lower depending on your calorie needs.

	Calories:	2,000	2,500
Total Fat	Less than	65g	80g
Sat Fat	Less than	20g	25g
Cholesterol	Less than	300mg	300mg
Sodium	Less than	2,400mg	2,400mg
Total Carbohydrate		300g	375g
Dietary Fiber		25g	30g

Start here

Check calories

Stick to 400-500 kcal per meal
200 kcal per snack

Quick guide to % DV

5% or less is low
20% or more is high

Limit these

Limit sodium to reduce blood pressure

Get enough of these

The body uses carbohydrates for energy, so still eat at least 45g carbs at each meal.
(If diabetic: Women 45g carbs max per meal
Men 60-75 g carbs per meal)

(Example Page)
Daily Weight Loss Planner

Date: __________

Calorie limit: 1400 kcal | fat limit: 40 g

TO DO LIST:

- pay cellphone bill

TODAY'S WEIGHT: 201 lb

TODAY'S WORKOUT WILL INCLUDE:

	TYPE:	DURATION:
☐ CARDIO:	EX: running, walking, biking, elliptical, etc.	30 mins
☐ RESISTANCE:	Push ups, sit ups, lunges, squats, weight lifting, etc	30 mins
☐ CLASS/OTHER	Yoga, Zumba, Body Combat etc.	60 mins

BREAKFAST   TIME: 7:00am

CARB: Breakfast potatoes

VEGGIE: Sauteed bellpeppers & onion

PROTEIN: Sauteed bellpeppers & onion

BEVERAGE: Water 8 oz

SNACK: 1/3 cup popcorn   TIME: 10:00 am

TOTAL CALORIES AT THIS MEAL: 400 kcal

TOTAL FAT AT THIS MEAL: 12 g

LUNCH

CARB: 1 baked sweet potato   TIME: 11:30 am

VEGGIE: 1 cup of broccoli

PROTEIN: 1 baked chicken breast

BEVERAGE:

SNACK: TIME:

TOTAL CALORIES AT THIS MEAL: 300 kcal

TOTAL FAT AT THIS MEAL: 8 g

DINNER   TIME:

CARB:

VEGGIE:

PROTEIN:

BEVERAGE:

SNACK: TIME:

TOTAL CALORIES AT THIS MEAL:

TOTAL FAT AT THIS MEAL:

HOW DID I DO TODAY?

TOTAL STEPS: 1600

STEP GOAL: 2000

TOTAL CALORIES CONSUMED: 700 kcal

TOTAL CALORIES BURNED: 400 kcal

TOTAL FAT CONSUMED: 20 g

TOTAL FAT BURNED: 13 g

Daily Weight Loss Planner

Date: Calorie limit: kcal | fat limit: g

TO DO LIST:

TODAY'S WORKOUT WILL INCLUDE:

TYPE: DURATION:

☐ CARDIO: __________ __________

☐ RESISTANCE: __________ __________

☐ CLASS/OTHER __________ __________

TODAY'S WEIGHT:

BREAKFAST

TIME:

CARB:

VEGGIE:

PROTEIN:

BEVERAGE:

SNACK: TIME:

TOTAL CALORIES AT THIS MEAL:

TOTAL FAT AT THIS MEAL:

LUNCH

TIME:

CARB:

VEGGIE:

PROTEIN:

BEVERAGE:

SNACK: TIME:

TOTAL CALORIES AT THIS MEAL:

TOTAL FAT AT THIS MEAL:

DINNER

TIME:

CARB:

VEGGIE:

PROTEIN:

BEVERAGE:

SNACK: TIME:

TOTAL CALORIES AT THIS MEAL:

TOTAL FAT AT THIS MEAL:

HOW DID I DO TODAY?

TOTAL STEPS:

STEP GOAL:

TOTAL CALORIES CONSUMED:

TOTAL CALORIES BURNED:

TOTAL FAT CONSUMED:

TOTAL FAT BURNED:

Daily Weight Loss Planner

Date: | Calorie limit: ___ kcal | fat limit: ___ g

TO DO LIST:

TODAY'S WORKOUT WILL INCLUDE:

	TYPE:	DURATION:
☐ CARDIO:	_____________	_____________
☐ RESISTANCE:	_____________	_____________
☐ CLASS/OTHER	_____________	_____________

TODAY'S WEIGHT:

BREAKFAST

CARB:

VEGGIE:

PROTEIN:

BEVERAGE:

SNACK:

TIME:

TOTAL CALORIES AT THIS MEAL:

TOTAL FAT AT THIS MEAL:

LUNCH

CARB:

VEGGIE:

PROTEIN:

BEVERAGE:

SNACK:

TIME:

TOTAL CALORIES AT THIS MEAL:

TOTAL FAT AT THIS MEAL:

DINNER

CARB:

VEGGIE:

PROTEIN:

BEVERAGE:

SNACK:

TIME:

TOTAL CALORIES AT THIS MEAL:

TOTAL FAT AT THIS MEAL:

HOW DID I DO TODAY?

TOTAL STEPS:

STEP GOAL:

TOTAL CALORIES CONSUMED:

TOTAL CALORIES BURNED:

TOTAL FAT CONSUMED:

TOTAL FAT BURNED:

Daily Weight Loss Planner

Date: Calorie limit: kcal | fat limit: g

TO DO LIST:

TODAY'S WORKOUT WILL INCLUDE:

TYPE: DURATION:

☐ CARDIO: _______________ _______________

☐ RESISTANCE: _______________ _______________

☐ CLASS/OTHER _______________ _______________

TODAY'S WEIGHT:

B R E A K F A S T   TIME:

CARB:

VEGGIE:

PROTEIN:

BEVERAGE:

SNACK: TIME:

TOTAL CALORIES AT THIS MEAL:

TOTAL FAT AT THIS MEAL:

L U N C H   TIME:

CARB:

VEGGIE:

PROTEIN:

BEVERAGE:

SNACK: TIME:

TOTAL CALORIES AT THIS MEAL:

TOTAL FAT AT THIS MEAL:

D I N N E R   TIME:

CARB:

VEGGIE:

PROTEIN:

BEVERAGE:

SNACK: TIME:

TOTAL CALORIES AT THIS MEAL:

TOTAL FAT AT THIS MEAL:

H O W D I D I D O TODAY?

TOTAL STEPS:

STEP GOAL:

TOTAL CALORIES CONSUMED:

TOTAL CALORIES BURNED:

TOTAL FAT CONSUMED:

TOTAL FAT BURNED:

Daily Weight Loss Planner

Date: Calorie limit: ____ kcal | fat limit: ____ g

TO DO LIST:

TODAY'S WEIGHT:

TODAY'S WORKOUT WILL INCLUDE:

TYPE: DURATION:

☐ CARDIO: ______________ ______________

☐ RESISTANCE: ______________ ______________

☐ CLASS/OTHER ______________ ______________

BREAKFAST

TIME: TOTAL CALORIES AT THIS MEAL: TOTAL FAT AT THIS MEAL:

CARB:

VEGGIE:

PROTEIN:

BEVERAGE:

SNACK: TIME:

LUNCH

TIME: TOTAL CALORIES AT THIS MEAL: TOTAL FAT AT THIS MEAL:

CARB:

VEGGIE:

PROTEIN:

BEVERAGE:

SNACK: TIME:

DINNER

TIME: TOTAL CALORIES AT THIS MEAL: TOTAL FAT AT THIS MEAL:

CARB:

VEGGIE:

PROTEIN:

BEVERAGE:

SNACK: TIME:

HOW DID I DO TODAY?

TOTAL STEPS: TOTAL CALORIES CONSUMED: TOTAL FAT CONSUMED:

STEP GOAL: TOTAL CALORIES BURNED: TOTAL FAT BURNED:

Daily Weight Loss Planner

Date: Calorie limit: kcal | fat limit: g

TO DO LIST:

TODAY'S WORKOUT WILL INCLUDE:

	TYPE:	DURATION:
☐ CARDIO:	_________	_________
☐ RESISTANCE:	_________	_________
☐ CLASS/OTHER	_________	_________

TODAY'S WEIGHT:

B R E A K F A S T   TIME:

CARB:

VEGGIE:

PROTEIN:

BEVERAGE:

SNACK: TIME:

TOTAL CALORIES AT THIS MEAL:	TOTAL FAT AT THIS MEAL:

L U N C H   TIME:

CARB:

VEGGIE:

PROTEIN:

BEVERAGE:

SNACK: TIME:

TOTAL CALORIES AT THIS MEAL:	TOTAL FAT AT THIS MEAL:

D I N N E R   TIME:

CARB:

VEGGIE:

PROTEIN:

BEVERAGE:

SNACK: TIME:

TOTAL CALORIES AT THIS MEAL:	TOTAL FAT AT THIS MEAL:

H O W   D I D   I   D O   T O D A Y?

TOTAL STEPS:

STEP GOAL:

TOTAL CALORIES CONSUMED:	TOTAL FAT CONSUMED:
TOTAL CALORIES BURNED:	TOTAL FAT BURNED:

Daily Weight Loss Planner

Date: Calorie limit: kcal | fat limit: g

TO DO LIST:

TODAY'S WORKOUT WILL INCLUDE:

	TYPE:	DURATION:
☐ CARDIO:	____________	____________
☐ RESISTANCE:	____________	____________
☐ CLASS/OTHER	____________	____________

TODAY'S WEIGHT:

B R E A K F A S T

TIME:

TOTAL CALORIES AT THIS MEAL:

TOTAL FAT AT THIS MEAL:

CARB:

VEGGIE:

PROTEIN:

BEVERAGE:

SNACK: TIME:

L U N C H

TIME:

TOTAL CALORIES AT THIS MEAL:

TOTAL FAT AT THIS MEAL:

CARB:

VEGGIE:

PROTEIN:

BEVERAGE:

SNACK: TIME:

D I N N E R

TIME:

TOTAL CALORIES AT THIS MEAL:

TOTAL FAT AT THIS MEAL:

CARB:

VEGGIE:

PROTEIN:

BEVERAGE:

SNACK: TIME:

H O W   D I D   I   D O   T O D A Y ?

TOTAL STEPS:

TOTAL CALORIES CONSUMED:

TOTAL FAT CONSUMED:

STEP GOAL:

TOTAL CALORIES BURNED:

TOTAL FAT BURNED:

Daily Weight Loss Planner

Date: ___________   Calorie limit: ______ kcal | fat limit: ___ g

TO DO LIST:

TODAY'S WORKOUT WILL INCLUDE:

TYPE: DURATION:

☐ CARDIO: _____________ _____________

☐ RESISTANCE: _____________ _____________

☐ CLASS/OTHER _____________ _____________

TODAY'S WEIGHT: ___________

BREAKFAST

TIME: _______

CARB:

VEGGIE:

PROTEIN:

BEVERAGE:

SNACK: TIME: _______

TOTAL CALORIES AT THIS MEAL:

TOTAL FAT AT THIS MEAL:

LUNCH

TIME: _______

CARB:

VEGGIE:

PROTEIN:

BEVERAGE:

SNACK: TIME: _______

TOTAL CALORIES AT THIS MEAL:

TOTAL FAT AT THIS MEAL:

DINNER

TIME: _______

CARB:

VEGGIE:

PROTEIN:

BEVERAGE:

SNACK: TIME: _______

TOTAL CALORIES AT THIS MEAL:

TOTAL FAT AT THIS MEAL:

HOW DID I DO TODAY?

TOTAL STEPS:

STEP GOAL:

TOTAL CALORIES CONSUMED:

TOTAL CALORIES BURNED:

TOTAL FAT CONSUMED:

TOTAL FAT BURNED:

Daily Weight Loss Planner

Date: **Calorie limit:**   kcal | **fat limit:**   g

TO DO LIST:

TODAY'S WORKOUT WILL INCLUDE:

TYPE: DURATION:

☐ CARDIO: _____________ _____________

☐ RESISTANCE: _____________ _____________

☐ CLASS/OTHER _____________ _____________

TODAY'S WEIGHT:

BREAKFAST

TIME:

CARB:

VEGGIE:

PROTEIN:

BEVERAGE:

SNACK: TIME:

TOTAL CALORIES AT THIS MEAL:

TOTAL FAT AT THIS MEAL:

LUNCH

TIME:

CARB:

VEGGIE:

PROTEIN:

BEVERAGE:

SNACK: TIME:

TOTAL CALORIES AT THIS MEAL:

TOTAL FAT AT THIS MEAL:

DINNER

TIME:

CARB:

VEGGIE:

PROTEIN:

BEVERAGE:

SNACK: TIME:

TOTAL CALORIES AT THIS MEAL:

TOTAL FAT AT THIS MEAL:

HOW DID I DO TODAY?

TOTAL STEPS:

STEP GOAL:

TOTAL CALORIES CONSUMED:

TOTAL CALORIES BURNED:

TOTAL FAT CONSUMED:

TOTAL FAT BURNED:

Daily Weight Loss Planner

Date: | Calorie limit: kcal | fat limit: g

TO DO LIST:

TODAY'S WORKOUT WILL INCLUDE:

TYPE: DURATION:

☐ CARDIO: _____________ _____________

☐ RESISTANCE: _____________ _____________

☐ CLASS/OTHER _____________ _____________

TODAY'S WEIGHT:

B R E A K F A S T
TIME:

TOTAL CALORIES AT THIS MEAL:

TOTAL FAT AT THIS MEAL:

CARB:

VEGGIE:

PROTEIN:

BEVERAGE:

SNACK: TIME:

L U N C H
TIME:

TOTAL CALORIES AT THIS MEAL:

TOTAL FAT AT THIS MEAL:

CARB:

VEGGIE:

PROTEIN:

BEVERAGE:

SNACK: TIME:

D I N N E R
TIME:

TOTAL CALORIES AT THIS MEAL:

TOTAL FAT AT THIS MEAL:

CARB:

VEGGIE:

PROTEIN:

BEVERAGE:

SNACK: TIME:

H O W   D I D   I   D O   TODAY?

TOTAL STEPS:

TOTAL CALORIES CONSUMED:

TOTAL FAT CONSUMED:

STEP GOAL:

TOTAL CALORIES BURNED:

TOTAL FAT BURNED:

Daily Weight Loss Planner

Date: _______________   Calorie limit: _______ kcal | fat limit: _______ g

TO DO LIST:

TODAY'S WORKOUT WILL INCLUDE:

	TYPE:	DURATION:
☐ CARDIO:	_______________	_______________
☐ RESISTANCE:	_______________	_______________
☐ CLASS/OTHER	_______________	_______________

TODAY'S WEIGHT:

B R E A K F A S T

TIME: _______

CARB:

VEGGIE:

PROTEIN:

BEVERAGE:

SNACK: _______ TIME: _______

TOTAL CALORIES AT THIS MEAL:

TOTAL FAT AT THIS MEAL:

L U N C H

TIME: _______

CARB:

VEGGIE:

PROTEIN:

BEVERAGE:

SNACK: _______ TIME: _______

TOTAL CALORIES AT THIS MEAL:

TOTAL FAT AT THIS MEAL:

D I N N E R

TIME: _______

CARB:

VEGGIE:

PROTEIN:

BEVERAGE:

SNACK: _______ TIME: _______

TOTAL CALORIES AT THIS MEAL:

TOTAL FAT AT THIS MEAL:

H O W   D I D   I   D O   T O D A Y?

TOTAL STEPS:

STEP GOAL:

TOTAL CALORIES CONSUMED:

TOTAL CALORIES BURNED:

TOTAL FAT CONSUMED:

TOTAL FAT BURNED:

Daily Weight Loss Planner

Date: Calorie limit: kcal | fat limit: g

TO DO LIST:

TODAY'S WEIGHT:

TODAY'S WORKOUT WILL INCLUDE:

TYPE: DURATION:

☐ CARDIO: _____________ _____________

☐ RESISTANCE: _____________ _____________

☐ CLASS/OTHER _____________ _____________

BREAKFAST

CARB:

VEGGIE:

PROTEIN:

BEVERAGE:

SNACK: TIME:

TIME:

TOTAL CALORIES AT THIS MEAL:

TOTAL FAT AT THIS MEAL:

LUNCH

CARB:

VEGGIE:

PROTEIN:

BEVERAGE:

SNACK: TIME:

TIME:

TOTAL CALORIES AT THIS MEAL:

TOTAL FAT AT THIS MEAL:

DINNER

CARB:

VEGGIE:

PROTEIN:

BEVERAGE:

SNACK: TIME:

TIME:

TOTAL CALORIES AT THIS MEAL:

TOTAL FAT AT THIS MEAL:

HOW DID I DO TODAY?

TOTAL STEPS:

STEP GOAL:

TOTAL CALORIES CONSUMED:

TOTAL CALORIES BURNED:

TOTAL FAT CONSUMED:

TOTAL FAT BURNED:

Daily Weight Loss Planner

Date: ___________ Calorie limit: _______ kcal | fat limit: _____ g

TO DO LIST:

TODAY'S WEIGHT:

TODAY'S WORKOUT WILL INCLUDE:

	TYPE:	DURATION:
☐ CARDIO:	______________	______________
☐ RESISTANCE:	______________	______________
☐ CLASS/OTHER	______________	______________

BREAKFAST

TIME: _______

CARB:

VEGGIE:

PROTEIN:

BEVERAGE:

SNACK: TIME:

TOTAL CALORIES AT THIS MEAL:

TOTAL FAT AT THIS MEAL:

LUNCH

TIME: _______

CARB:

VEGGIE:

PROTEIN:

BEVERAGE:

SNACK: TIME:

TOTAL CALORIES AT THIS MEAL:

TOTAL FAT AT THIS MEAL:

DINNER

TIME: _______

CARB:

VEGGIE:

PROTEIN:

BEVERAGE:

SNACK: TIME:

TOTAL CALORIES AT THIS MEAL:

TOTAL FAT AT THIS MEAL:

HOW DID I DO TODAY?

TOTAL STEPS:

STEP GOAL:

TOTAL CALORIES CONSUMED:

TOTAL CALORIES BURNED:

TOTAL FAT CONSUMED:

TOTAL FAT BURNED:

Daily Weight Loss Planner

Date: Calorie limit: kcal | fat limit: g

TO DO LIST:

TODAY'S WORKOUT WILL INCLUDE:

TYPE: DURATION:

☐ CARDIO: _______________ _______________

☐ RESISTANCE: _______________ _______________

☐ CLASS/OTHER _______________ _______________

TODAY'S WEIGHT:

BREAKFAST

TIME:

CARB:

VEGGIE:

PROTEIN:

BEVERAGE:

SNACK: TIME:

TOTAL CALORIES AT THIS MEAL:

TOTAL FAT AT THIS MEAL:

LUNCH

TIME:

CARB:

VEGGIE:

PROTEIN:

BEVERAGE:

SNACK: TIME:

TOTAL CALORIES AT THIS MEAL:

TOTAL FAT AT THIS MEAL:

DINNER

TIME:

CARB:

VEGGIE:

PROTEIN:

BEVERAGE:

SNACK: TIME:

TOTAL CALORIES AT THIS MEAL:

TOTAL FAT AT THIS MEAL:

HOW DID I DO TODAY?

TOTAL STEPS:

STEP GOAL:

TOTAL CALORIES CONSUMED:

TOTAL CALORIES BURNED:

TOTAL FAT CONSUMED:

TOTAL FAT BURNED:

Daily Weight Loss Planner

Date: ___________ **Calorie limit:** _____ kcal | **fat limit:** _____ g

TO DO LIST:

TODAY'S WEIGHT:

TODAY'S WORKOUT WILL INCLUDE:

	TYPE:	DURATION:
☐ CARDIO:	______________	______________
☐ RESISTANCE:	______________	______________
☐ CLASS/OTHER	______________	______________

BREAKFAST

TIME: _______

CARB:

VEGGIE:

PROTEIN:

BEVERAGE:

SNACK: TIME: _______

TOTAL CALORIES AT THIS MEAL:

TOTAL FAT AT THIS MEAL:

LUNCH

TIME: _______

CARB:

VEGGIE:

PROTEIN:

BEVERAGE:

SNACK: TIME: _______

TOTAL CALORIES AT THIS MEAL:

TOTAL FAT AT THIS MEAL:

DINNER

TIME: _______

CARB:

VEGGIE:

PROTEIN:

BEVERAGE:

SNACK: TIME: _______

TOTAL CALORIES AT THIS MEAL:

TOTAL FAT AT THIS MEAL:

HOW DID I DO TODAY?

TOTAL STEPS:

STEP GOAL:

TOTAL CALORIES CONSUMED:

TOTAL CALORIES BURNED:

TOTAL FAT CONSUMED:

TOTAL FAT BURNED:

Daily Weight Loss Planner

Date: _______________   Calorie limit: _______ kcal | fat limit: _______ g

TO DO LIST:

TODAY'S WORKOUT WILL INCLUDE:

	TYPE:	DURATION:
☐ CARDIO:	_____________	_____________
☐ RESISTANCE:	_____________	_____________
☐ CLASS/OTHER	_____________	_____________

TODAY'S WEIGHT: _______________

BREAKFAST   TIME: _______

CARB:

VEGGIE:

PROTEIN:

BEVERAGE:

SNACK: TIME: _______

TOTAL CALORIES AT THIS MEAL:

TOTAL FAT AT THIS MEAL:

LUNCH   TIME: _______

CARB:

VEGGIE:

PROTEIN:

BEVERAGE:

SNACK: TIME: _______

TOTAL CALORIES AT THIS MEAL:

TOTAL FAT AT THIS MEAL:

DINNER   TIME: _______

CARB:

VEGGIE:

PROTEIN:

BEVERAGE:

SNACK: TIME: _______

TOTAL CALORIES AT THIS MEAL:

TOTAL FAT AT THIS MEAL:

HOW DID I DO TODAY?

TOTAL STEPS:

STEP GOAL:

TOTAL CALORIES CONSUMED:

TOTAL CALORIES BURNED:

TOTAL FAT CONSUMED:

TOTAL FAT BURNED:

Daily Weight Loss Planner

Date: ___________________   Calorie limit: _______ kcal | fat limit: _______ g

---

TO DO LIST:

TODAY'S WEIGHT:

TODAY'S WORKOUT WILL INCLUDE:

	TYPE:	DURATION:
☐ CARDIO:	___________	___________
☐ RESISTANCE:	___________	___________
☐ CLASS/OTHER	___________	___________

BREAKFAST   TIME: ___

CARB:

VEGGIE:

PROTEIN:

BEVERAGE:

SNACK: TIME: ___

TOTAL CALORIES AT THIS MEAL:	TOTAL FAT AT THIS MEAL:

LUNCH   TIME: ___

CARB:

VEGGIE:

PROTEIN:

BEVERAGE:

SNACK: TIME: ___

TOTAL CALORIES AT THIS MEAL:	TOTAL FAT AT THIS MEAL:

DINNER   TIME: ___

CARB:

VEGGIE:

PROTEIN:

BEVERAGE:

SNACK: TIME: ___

TOTAL CALORIES AT THIS MEAL:	TOTAL FAT AT THIS MEAL:

HOW DID I DO TODAY?

TOTAL STEPS:	TOTAL CALORIES CONSUMED:	TOTAL FAT CONSUMED:
STEP GOAL:	TOTAL CALORIES BURNED:	TOTAL FAT BURNED:

Daily Weight Loss Planner

Date: Calorie limit: kcal | fat limit: g

TO DO LIST:

TODAY'S WORKOUT WILL INCLUDE:

TYPE: DURATION:

☐ CARDIO: ______________ ______________

☐ RESISTANCE: ______________ ______________

☐ CLASS/OTHER ______________ ______________

TODAY'S WEIGHT:

B R E A K F A S T

TIME:

CARB:

VEGGIE:

PROTEIN:

BEVERAGE:

SNACK: TIME:

TOTAL CALORIES AT THIS MEAL:

TOTAL FAT AT THIS MEAL:

L U N C H

TIME:

CARB:

VEGGIE:

PROTEIN:

BEVERAGE:

SNACK: TIME:

TOTAL CALORIES AT THIS MEAL:

TOTAL FAT AT THIS MEAL:

D I N N E R

TIME:

CARB:

VEGGIE:

PROTEIN:

BEVERAGE:

SNACK: TIME:

TOTAL CALORIES AT THIS MEAL:

TOTAL FAT AT THIS MEAL:

H O W   D I D   I   D O   TODAY?

TOTAL STEPS:

STEP GOAL:

TOTAL CALORIES CONSUMED:

TOTAL CALORIES BURNED:

TOTAL FAT CONSUMED:

TOTAL FAT BURNED:

Daily Weight Loss Planner

Date: ____________   Calorie limit: ______ kcal | fat limit: ______ g

TO DO LIST:

TODAY'S WORKOUT WILL INCLUDE:

TYPE: DURATION:

☐ CARDIO: ____________ ____________

☐ RESISTANCE: ____________ ____________

☐ CLASS/OTHER ____________ ____________

TODAY'S WEIGHT: ____________

BREAKFAST

TIME: ____________

CARB:

VEGGIE:

PROTEIN:

BEVERAGE:

SNACK: TIME: ____________

TOTAL CALORIES AT THIS MEAL:

TOTAL FAT AT THIS MEAL:

LUNCH

TIME: ____________

CARB:

VEGGIE:

PROTEIN:

BEVERAGE:

SNACK: TIME: ____________

TOTAL CALORIES AT THIS MEAL:

TOTAL FAT AT THIS MEAL:

DINNER

TIME: ____________

CARB:

VEGGIE:

PROTEIN:

BEVERAGE:

SNACK: TIME: ____________

TOTAL CALORIES AT THIS MEAL:

TOTAL FAT AT THIS MEAL:

HOW DID I DO TODAY?

TOTAL STEPS:

STEP GOAL:

TOTAL CALORIES CONSUMED:

TOTAL CALORIES BURNED:

TOTAL FAT CONSUMED:

TOTAL FAT BURNED:

Daily Weight Loss Planner

| Date: | Calorie limit: ______ kcal | fat limit: ______ g |

TO DO LIST:

TODAY'S WORKOUT WILL INCLUDE:

	TYPE:	DURATION:
☐ CARDIO:	______________	______________
☐ RESISTANCE:	______________	______________
☐ CLASS/OTHER	______________	______________

TODAY'S WEIGHT:

BREAKFAST

TIME:

CARB:

VEGGIE:

PROTEIN:

BEVERAGE:

SNACK: TIME:

TOTAL CALORIES AT THIS MEAL:

TOTAL FAT AT THIS MEAL:

LUNCH

TIME:

CARB:

VEGGIE:

PROTEIN:

BEVERAGE:

SNACK: TIME:

TOTAL CALORIES AT THIS MEAL:

TOTAL FAT AT THIS MEAL:

DINNER

TIME:

CARB:

VEGGIE:

PROTEIN:

BEVERAGE:

SNACK: TIME:

TOTAL CALORIES AT THIS MEAL:

TOTAL FAT AT THIS MEAL:

HOW DID I DO TODAY?

TOTAL STEPS:

STEP GOAL:

TOTAL CALORIES CONSUMED:

TOTAL CALORIES BURNED:

TOTAL FAT CONSUMED:

TOTAL FAT BURNED:

Daily Weight Loss Planner

Date: ___________ **Calorie limit:** ___ kcal | **fat limit:** ___ g

TO DO LIST:

TODAY'S WEIGHT:

TODAY'S WORKOUT WILL INCLUDE:

	TYPE:	DURATION:
☐ CARDIO:	___________	___________
☐ RESISTANCE:	___________	___________
☐ CLASS/OTHER	___________	___________

BREAKFAST

TIME: ___

CARB:

VEGGIE:

PROTEIN:

BEVERAGE:

SNACK: TIME: ___

TOTAL CALORIES AT THIS MEAL:

TOTAL FAT AT THIS MEAL:

LUNCH

TIME: ___

CARB:

VEGGIE:

PROTEIN:

BEVERAGE:

SNACK: TIME: ___

TOTAL CALORIES AT THIS MEAL:

TOTAL FAT AT THIS MEAL:

DINNER

TIME: ___

CARB:

VEGGIE:

PROTEIN:

BEVERAGE:

SNACK: TIME: ___

TOTAL CALORIES AT THIS MEAL:

TOTAL FAT AT THIS MEAL:

HOW DID I DO TODAY?

TOTAL STEPS:

STEP GOAL:

TOTAL CALORIES CONSUMED:

TOTAL CALORIES BURNED:

TOTAL FAT CONSUMED:

TOTAL FAT BURNED:

Daily Weight Loss Planner

Date: __________________   Calorie limit: __________ kcal | fat limit: __________ g

TO DO LIST:

TODAY'S WORKOUT WILL INCLUDE:

	TYPE:	DURATION:
☐ CARDIO:	_____________	_____________
☐ RESISTANCE:	_____________	_____________
☐ CLASS/OTHER	_____________	_____________

TODAY'S WEIGHT:

BREAKFAST
TIME:

CARB:

VEGGIE:

PROTEIN:

BEVERAGE:

SNACK: TIME:

TOTAL CALORIES AT THIS MEAL:

TOTAL FAT AT THIS MEAL:

LUNCH
TIME:

CARB:

VEGGIE:

PROTEIN:

BEVERAGE:

SNACK: TIME:

TOTAL CALORIES AT THIS MEAL:

TOTAL FAT AT THIS MEAL:

DINNER
TIME:

CARB:

VEGGIE:

PROTEIN:

BEVERAGE:

SNACK: TIME:

TOTAL CALORIES AT THIS MEAL:

TOTAL FAT AT THIS MEAL:

HOW DID I DO TODAY?

TOTAL STEPS:

STEP GOAL:

TOTAL CALORIES CONSUMED:

TOTAL CALORIES BURNED:

TOTAL FAT CONSUMED:

TOTAL FAT BURNED:

Daily Weight Loss Planner

Date: ______________________   Calorie limit: ______ kcal | fat limit: ______ g

TO DO LIST:

TODAY'S WEIGHT:

TODAY'S WORKOUT WILL INCLUDE:

TYPE: DURATION:

☐ CARDIO: ______________ ______________

☐ RESISTANCE: ______________ ______________

☐ CLASS/OTHER ______________ ______________

BREAKFAST

TIME:

CARB:

VEGGIE:

PROTEIN:

BEVERAGE:

SNACK: TIME:

TOTAL CALORIES AT THIS MEAL:

TOTAL FAT AT THIS MEAL:

LUNCH

TIME:

CARB:

VEGGIE:

PROTEIN:

BEVERAGE:

SNACK: TIME:

TOTAL CALORIES AT THIS MEAL:

TOTAL FAT AT THIS MEAL:

DINNER

TIME:

CARB:

VEGGIE:

PROTEIN:

BEVERAGE:

SNACK: TIME:

TOTAL CALORIES AT THIS MEAL:

TOTAL FAT AT THIS MEAL:

HOW DID I DO TODAY?

TOTAL STEPS:

STEP GOAL:

TOTAL CALORIES CONSUMED:

TOTAL CALORIES BURNED:

TOTAL FAT CONSUMED:

TOTAL FAT BURNED:

Daily Weight Loss Planner

Date: | Calorie limit: ___ kcal | fat limit: ___ g

TO DO LIST:

TODAY'S WORKOUT WILL INCLUDE:

TYPE: DURATION:

☐ CARDIO: _____________ _____________

☐ RESISTANCE: _____________ _____________

☐ CLASS/OTHER _____________ _____________

TODAY'S WEIGHT:

BREAKFAST   TIME:

CARB:

VEGGIE:

PROTEIN:

BEVERAGE:

SNACK: TIME:

TOTAL CALORIES AT THIS MEAL:

TOTAL FAT AT THIS MEAL:

LUNCH   TIME:

CARB:

VEGGIE:

PROTEIN:

BEVERAGE:

SNACK: TIME:

TOTAL CALORIES AT THIS MEAL:

TOTAL FAT AT THIS MEAL:

DINNER   TIME:

CARB:

VEGGIE:

PROTEIN:

BEVERAGE:

SNACK: TIME:

TOTAL CALORIES AT THIS MEAL:

TOTAL FAT AT THIS MEAL:

HOW DID I DO TODAY?

TOTAL STEPS:

STEP GOAL:

TOTAL CALORIES CONSUMED:

TOTAL CALORIES BURNED:

TOTAL FAT CONSUMED:

TOTAL FAT BURNED:

Daily Weight Loss Planner

Date: ___________   Calorie limit: _______ kcal | fat limit: _______ g

---

TO DO LIST:

TODAY'S WORKOUT WILL INCLUDE:

	TYPE:	DURATION:
☐ CARDIO:	_____________	_____________
☐ RESISTANCE:	_____________	_____________
☐ CLASS/OTHER	_____________	_____________

TODAY'S WEIGHT: _______

B R E A K F A S T   TIME: _______

CARB:

VEGGIE:

PROTEIN:

BEVERAGE:

SNACK: TIME: _______

TOTAL CALORIES AT THIS MEAL:	TOTAL FAT AT THIS MEAL:

L U N C H   TIME: _______

CARB:

VEGGIE:

PROTEIN:

BEVERAGE:

SNACK: TIME: _______

TOTAL CALORIES AT THIS MEAL:	TOTAL FAT AT THIS MEAL:

D I N N E R   TIME: _______

CARB:

VEGGIE:

PROTEIN:

BEVERAGE:

SNACK: TIME: _______

TOTAL CALORIES AT THIS MEAL:	TOTAL FAT AT THIS MEAL:

H O W   D I D   I   D O   T O D A Y ?

	TOTAL CALORIES CONSUMED:	TOTAL FAT CONSUMED:
TOTAL STEPS:		
STEP GOAL:	TOTAL CALORIES BURNED:	TOTAL FAT BURNED:

Daily Weight Loss Planner

Date: Calorie limit: kcal | fat limit: g

TO DO LIST:

TODAY'S WEIGHT:

TODAY'S WORKOUT WILL INCLUDE:

TYPE: DURATION:

☐ CARDIO: _____________ _____________

☐ RESISTANCE: _____________ _____________

☐ CLASS/OTHER _____________ _____________

BREAKFAST

TIME:

CARB:

VEGGIE:

PROTEIN:

BEVERAGE:

SNACK: TIME:

TOTAL CALORIES AT THIS MEAL:

TOTAL FAT AT THIS MEAL:

LUNCH

TIME:

CARB:

VEGGIE:

PROTEIN:

BEVERAGE:

SNACK: TIME:

TOTAL CALORIES AT THIS MEAL:

TOTAL FAT AT THIS MEAL:

DINNER

TIME:

CARB:

VEGGIE:

PROTEIN:

BEVERAGE:

SNACK: TIME:

TOTAL CALORIES AT THIS MEAL:

TOTAL FAT AT THIS MEAL:

HOW DID I DO TODAY?

TOTAL STEPS:

STEP GOAL:

TOTAL CALORIES CONSUMED:

TOTAL CALORIES BURNED:

TOTAL FAT CONSUMED:

TOTAL FAT BURNED:

Daily Weight Loss Planner

Date: _______________   Calorie limit: ______ kcal | fat limit: ______ g

TO DO LIST:

TODAY'S WEIGHT:

TODAY'S WORKOUT WILL INCLUDE:

	TYPE:	DURATION:
☐ CARDIO:	_____________	_____________
☐ RESISTANCE:	_____________	_____________
☐ CLASS/OTHER	_____________	_____________

BREAKFAST

TIME:

CARB:

VEGGIE:

PROTEIN:

BEVERAGE:

SNACK: TIME:

TOTAL CALORIES AT THIS MEAL:

TOTAL FAT AT THIS MEAL:

LUNCH

TIME:

CARB:

VEGGIE:

PROTEIN:

BEVERAGE:

SNACK: TIME:

TOTAL CALORIES AT THIS MEAL:

TOTAL FAT AT THIS MEAL:

DINNER

TIME:

CARB:

VEGGIE:

PROTEIN:

BEVERAGE:

SNACK: TIME:

TOTAL CALORIES AT THIS MEAL:

TOTAL FAT AT THIS MEAL:

HOW DID I DO TODAY?

TOTAL STEPS:

STEP GOAL:

TOTAL CALORIES CONSUMED:

TOTAL CALORIES BURNED:

TOTAL FAT CONSUMED:

TOTAL FAT BURNED:

Daily Weight Loss Planner

Date: | **Calorie limit:** kcal | **fat limit:** g

TO DO LIST:

TODAY'S WEIGHT:

TODAY'S WORKOUT WILL INCLUDE:

TYPE: | DURATION:

☐ CARDIO: _____________ _____________

☐ RESISTANCE: _____________ _____________

☐ CLASS/OTHER _____________ _____________

BREAKFAST

TIME:

CARB:

VEGGIE:

PROTEIN:

BEVERAGE:

SNACK: TIME:

TOTAL CALORIES AT THIS MEAL:

TOTAL FAT AT THIS MEAL:

LUNCH

TIME:

CARB:

VEGGIE:

PROTEIN:

BEVERAGE:

SNACK: TIME:

TOTAL CALORIES AT THIS MEAL:

TOTAL FAT AT THIS MEAL:

DINNER

TIME:

CARB:

VEGGIE:

PROTEIN:

BEVERAGE:

SNACK: TIME:

TOTAL CALORIES AT THIS MEAL:

TOTAL FAT AT THIS MEAL:

HOW DID I DO TODAY?

TOTAL STEPS:

STEP GOAL:

TOTAL CALORIES CONSUMED:

TOTAL CALORIES BURNED:

TOTAL FAT CONSUMED:

TOTAL FAT BURNED:

Daily Weight Loss Planner

D a t e : | Calorie limit: _____ kcal | fat limit: _____ g

TO DO LIST:

TODAY'S WEIGHT:

TODAY'S WORKOUT WILL INCLUDE:

	TYPE:	DURATION:
☐ CARDIO:	_____________	_____________
☐ RESISTANCE:	_____________	_____________
☐ CLASS/OTHER	_____________	_____________

B R E A K F A S T

TIME:

CARB:

VEGGIE:

PROTEIN:

BEVERAGE:

SNACK: TIME:

TOTAL CALORIES AT THIS MEAL:

TOTAL FAT AT THIS MEAL:

L U N C H

TIME:

CARB:

VEGGIE:

PROTEIN:

BEVERAGE:

SNACK: TIME:

TOTAL CALORIES AT THIS MEAL:

TOTAL FAT AT THIS MEAL:

D I N N E R

TIME:

CARB:

VEGGIE:

PROTEIN:

BEVERAGE:

SNACK: TIME:

TOTAL CALORIES AT THIS MEAL:

TOTAL FAT AT THIS MEAL:

H O W   D I D   I   D O   TODAY?

TOTAL STEPS:

STEP GOAL:

TOTAL CALORIES CONSUMED:

TOTAL CALORIES BURNED:

TOTAL FAT CONSUMED:

TOTAL FAT BURNED:

Daily Weight Loss Planner

Date: Calorie limit: kcal | fat limit: g

TO DO LIST:

TODAY'S WORKOUT WILL INCLUDE:

                                                TYPE: DURATION:

☐ CARDIO: ___________ ___________

☐ RESISTANCE: ___________ ___________

☐ CLASS/OTHER ___________ ___________

TODAY'S WEIGHT:

BREAKFAST   TIME:

CARB:

VEGGIE:

PROTEIN:

BEVERAGE:

SNACK: TIME:

TOTAL CALORIES AT THIS MEAL:

TOTAL FAT AT THIS MEAL:

LUNCH   TIME:

CARB:

VEGGIE:

PROTEIN:

BEVERAGE:

SNACK: TIME:

TOTAL CALORIES AT THIS MEAL:

TOTAL FAT AT THIS MEAL:

DINNER   TIME:

CARB:

VEGGIE:

PROTEIN:

BEVERAGE:

SNACK: TIME:

TOTAL CALORIES AT THIS MEAL:

TOTAL FAT AT THIS MEAL:

HOW DID I DO TODAY?

TOTAL STEPS:

STEP GOAL:

TOTAL CALORIES CONSUMED:

TOTAL CALORIES BURNED:

TOTAL FAT CONSUMED:

TOTAL FAT BURNED:

Daily Weight Loss Planner

Date: | Calorie limit: ______ kcal | fat limit: ______ g

TO DO LIST:

TODAY'S WEIGHT:

TODAY'S WORKOUT WILL INCLUDE:

	TYPE:	DURATION:
☐ CARDIO:	______________	______________
☐ RESISTANCE:	______________	______________
☐ CLASS/OTHER	______________	______________

BREAKFAST

TIME: ________ | TOTAL CALORIES AT THIS MEAL: | TOTAL FAT AT THIS MEAL:

CARB:

VEGGIE:

PROTEIN:

BEVERAGE:

SNACK: TIME: ________

LUNCH

TIME: ________ | TOTAL CALORIES AT THIS MEAL: | TOTAL FAT AT THIS MEAL:

CARB:

VEGGIE:

PROTEIN:

BEVERAGE:

SNACK: TIME: ________

DINNER

TIME: ________ | TOTAL CALORIES AT THIS MEAL: | TOTAL FAT AT THIS MEAL:

CARB:

VEGGIE:

PROTEIN:

BEVERAGE:

SNACK: TIME: ________

HOW DID I DO TODAY?

TOTAL STEPS: | TOTAL CALORIES CONSUMED: | TOTAL FAT CONSUMED:

STEP GOAL: | TOTAL CALORIES BURNED: | TOTAL FAT BURNED:

Daily Weight Loss Planner

Date: Calorie limit: kcal | fat limit: g

TO DO LIST:

TODAY'S WORKOUT WILL INCLUDE:

TYPE: DURATION:

☐ CARDIO: _____________ _____________

☐ RESISTANCE: _____________ _____________

☐ CLASS/OTHER _____________ _____________

TODAY'S WEIGHT:

BREAKFAST

TIME:

TOTAL CALORIES AT THIS MEAL:

TOTAL FAT AT THIS MEAL:

CARB:

VEGGIE:

PROTEIN:

BEVERAGE:

SNACK: TIME:

LUNCH

TIME:

TOTAL CALORIES AT THIS MEAL:

TOTAL FAT AT THIS MEAL:

CARB:

VEGGIE:

PROTEIN:

BEVERAGE:

SNACK: TIME:

DINNER

TIME:

TOTAL CALORIES AT THIS MEAL:

TOTAL FAT AT THIS MEAL:

CARB:

VEGGIE:

PROTEIN:

BEVERAGE:

SNACK: TIME:

HOW DID I DO TODAY?

TOTAL STEPS:

TOTAL CALORIES CONSUMED:

TOTAL FAT CONSUMED:

STEP GOAL:

TOTAL CALORIES BURNED:

TOTAL FAT BURNED:

Daily Weight Loss Planner

Date: Calorie limit: kcal | fat limit: g

TO DO LIST:

TODAY'S WORKOUT WILL INCLUDE:

TYPE: DURATION:

☐ CARDIO: ______________ ______________

☐ RESISTANCE: ______________ ______________

☐ CLASS/OTHER ______________ ______________

TODAY'S WEIGHT:

BREAKFAST

TIME:

TOTAL CALORIES AT THIS MEAL:

TOTAL FAT AT THIS MEAL:

CARB:

VEGGIE:

PROTEIN:

BEVERAGE:

SNACK: TIME:

LUNCH

TIME:

TOTAL CALORIES AT THIS MEAL:

TOTAL FAT AT THIS MEAL:

CARB:

VEGGIE:

PROTEIN:

BEVERAGE:

SNACK: TIME:

DINNER

TIME:

TOTAL CALORIES AT THIS MEAL:

TOTAL FAT AT THIS MEAL:

CARB:

VEGGIE:

PROTEIN:

BEVERAGE:

SNACK: TIME:

HOW DID I DO TODAY?

TOTAL STEPS:

TOTAL CALORIES CONSUMED:

TOTAL FAT CONSUMED:

STEP GOAL:

TOTAL CALORIES BURNED:

TOTAL FAT BURNED:

Daily Weight Loss Planner

Date: Calorie limit: kcal | fat limit: g

TO DO LIST:

TODAY'S WEIGHT:

TODAY'S WORKOUT WILL INCLUDE:

	TYPE:	DURATION:
☐ CARDIO:	_____________	_____________
☐ RESISTANCE:	_____________	_____________
☐ CLASS/OTHER	_____________	_____________

BREAKFAST

TIME:

CARB:

VEGGIE:

PROTEIN:

BEVERAGE:

SNACK: TIME:

TOTAL CALORIES AT THIS MEAL:

TOTAL FAT AT THIS MEAL:

LUNCH

TIME:

CARB:

VEGGIE:

PROTEIN:

BEVERAGE:

SNACK: TIME:

TOTAL CALORIES AT THIS MEAL:

TOTAL FAT AT THIS MEAL:

DINNER

TIME:

CARB:

VEGGIE:

PROTEIN:

BEVERAGE:

SNACK: TIME:

TOTAL CALORIES AT THIS MEAL:

TOTAL FAT AT THIS MEAL:

HOW DID I DO TODAY?

TOTAL STEPS:

STEP GOAL:

TOTAL CALORIES CONSUMED:

TOTAL CALORIES BURNED:

TOTAL FAT CONSUMED:

TOTAL FAT BURNED:

Daily Weight Loss Planner

Date: ______________ Calorie limit: ______ kcal | fat limit: ______ g

---

TO DO LIST:

TODAY'S WORKOUT WILL INCLUDE:

	TYPE:	DURATION:
☐ CARDIO:	______________	______________
☐ RESISTANCE:	______________	______________
☐ CLASS/OTHER	______________	______________

TODAY'S WEIGHT:

BREAKFAST TIME: ______

CARB:

VEGGIE:

PROTEIN:

BEVERAGE:

SNACK: TIME: ______

TOTAL CALORIES AT THIS MEAL:

TOTAL FAT AT THIS MEAL:

LUNCH TIME: ______

CARB:

VEGGIE:

PROTEIN:

BEVERAGE:

SNACK: TIME: ______

TOTAL CALORIES AT THIS MEAL:

TOTAL FAT AT THIS MEAL:

DINNER TIME: ______

CARB:

VEGGIE:

PROTEIN:

BEVERAGE:

SNACK: TIME: ______

TOTAL CALORIES AT THIS MEAL:

TOTAL FAT AT THIS MEAL:

HOW DID I DO TODAY?

TOTAL STEPS:

STEP GOAL:

TOTAL CALORIES CONSUMED:

TOTAL CALORIES BURNED:

TOTAL FAT CONSUMED:

TOTAL FAT BURNED:

Daily Weight Loss Planner

Date: | Calorie limit: kcal | fat limit: g

TO DO LIST:

TODAY'S WEIGHT:

TODAY'S WORKOUT WILL INCLUDE:

TYPE: | DURATION:

☐ CARDIO: _____________ _____________

☐ RESISTANCE: _____________ _____________

☐ CLASS/OTHER _____________ _____________

BREAKFAST

TIME:

CARB:

VEGGIE:

PROTEIN:

BEVERAGE:

SNACK: | TIME:

TOTAL CALORIES AT THIS MEAL:

TOTAL FAT AT THIS MEAL:

LUNCH

TIME:

CARB:

VEGGIE:

PROTEIN:

BEVERAGE:

SNACK: | TIME:

TOTAL CALORIES AT THIS MEAL:

TOTAL FAT AT THIS MEAL:

DINNER

TIME:

CARB:

VEGGIE:

PROTEIN:

BEVERAGE:

SNACK: | TIME:

TOTAL CALORIES AT THIS MEAL:

TOTAL FAT AT THIS MEAL:

HOW DID I DO TODAY?

TOTAL STEPS:

STEP GOAL:

TOTAL CALORIES CONSUMED:

TOTAL CALORIES BURNED:

TOTAL FAT CONSUMED:

TOTAL FAT BURNED:

Daily Weight Loss Planner

Date: ___________________

Calorie limit: ________ kcal | fat limit: ________ g

TO DO LIST:

TODAY'S WORKOUT WILL INCLUDE:

TYPE: DURATION:

☐ CARDIO: ______________ ______________

☐ RESISTANCE: ______________ ______________

☐ CLASS/OTHER ______________ ______________

TODAY'S WEIGHT:

B R E A K F A S T

TIME:

CARB:

VEGGIE:

PROTEIN:

BEVERAGE:

SNACK: TIME:

TOTAL CALORIES AT THIS MEAL:

TOTAL FAT AT THIS MEAL:

L U N C H

TIME:

CARB:

VEGGIE:

PROTEIN:

BEVERAGE:

SNACK: TIME:

TOTAL CALORIES AT THIS MEAL:

TOTAL FAT AT THIS MEAL:

D I N N E R

TIME:

CARB:

VEGGIE:

PROTEIN:

BEVERAGE:

SNACK: TIME:

TOTAL CALORIES AT THIS MEAL:

TOTAL FAT AT THIS MEAL:

H O W   D I D   I   D O   T O D A Y ?

TOTAL STEPS:

STEP GOAL:

TOTAL CALORIES CONSUMED:

TOTAL CALORIES BURNED:

TOTAL FAT CONSUMED:

TOTAL FAT BURNED:

Daily Weight Loss Planner

D a t e :   Calorie limit: kcal | fat limit: g

TO DO LIST:

TODAY'S WORKOUT WILL INCLUDE:

TYPE: DURATION:

☐ **CARDIO:** __________ __________

☐ **RESISTANCE:** __________ __________

TODAY'S WEIGHT:

☐ **CLASS/OTHER** __________ __________

B R E A K F A S T

TIME:

TOTAL CALORIES AT THIS MEAL:

TOTAL FAT AT THIS MEAL:

CARB:

VEGGIE:

PROTEIN:

BEVERAGE:

SNACK: TIME:

L U N C H

TIME:

TOTAL CALORIES AT THIS MEAL:

TOTAL FAT AT THIS MEAL:

CARB:

VEGGIE:

PROTEIN:

BEVERAGE:

SNACK: TIME:

D I N N E R

TIME:

TOTAL CALORIES AT THIS MEAL:

TOTAL FAT AT THIS MEAL:

CARB:

VEGGIE:

PROTEIN:

BEVERAGE:

SNACK: TIME:

H O W   D I D   I   D O   TODAY?

TOTAL STEPS:

TOTAL CALORIES CONSUMED:

TOTAL FAT CONSUMED:

STEP GOAL:

TOTAL CALORIES BURNED:

TOTAL FAT BURNED:

Daily Weight Loss Planner

Date: ___________ Calorie limit: ______ kcal | fat limit: ______ g

TO DO LIST:

TODAY'S WEIGHT:

TODAY'S WORKOUT WILL INCLUDE:

	TYPE:	DURATION:
☐ CARDIO:	___________	___________
☐ RESISTANCE:	___________	___________
☐ CLASS/OTHER	___________	___________

BREAKFAST

TIME: ______

CARB:

VEGGIE:

PROTEIN:

BEVERAGE:

SNACK: TIME: ______

TOTAL CALORIES AT THIS MEAL:

TOTAL FAT AT THIS MEAL:

LUNCH

TIME: ______

CARB:

VEGGIE:

PROTEIN:

BEVERAGE:

SNACK: TIME: ______

TOTAL CALORIES AT THIS MEAL:

TOTAL FAT AT THIS MEAL:

DINNER

TIME: ______

CARB:

VEGGIE:

PROTEIN:

BEVERAGE:

SNACK: TIME: ______

TOTAL CALORIES AT THIS MEAL:

TOTAL FAT AT THIS MEAL:

HOW DID I DO TODAY?

TOTAL STEPS:

STEP GOAL:

TOTAL CALORIES CONSUMED:

TOTAL CALORIES BURNED:

TOTAL FAT CONSUMED:

TOTAL FAT BURNED:

Daily Weight Loss Planner

<table>
<tr><td>Date:</td><td colspan="2">Calorie limit: kcal | fat limit: g</td></tr>
</table>

TO DO LIST:

TODAY'S WORKOUT WILL INCLUDE:

	TYPE:	DURATION:
☐ CARDIO:	___________	___________
☐ RESISTANCE:	___________	___________
☐ CLASS/OTHER	___________	___________

TODAY'S WEIGHT:

BREAKFAST

TIME:

CARB:

VEGGIE:

PROTEIN:

BEVERAGE:

SNACK: TIME:

TOTAL CALORIES AT THIS MEAL:

TOTAL FAT AT THIS MEAL:

LUNCH

TIME:

CARB:

VEGGIE:

PROTEIN:

BEVERAGE:

SNACK: TIME:

TOTAL CALORIES AT THIS MEAL:

TOTAL FAT AT THIS MEAL:

DINNER

TIME:

CARB:

VEGGIE:

PROTEIN:

BEVERAGE:

SNACK: TIME:

TOTAL CALORIES AT THIS MEAL:

TOTAL FAT AT THIS MEAL:

HOW DID I DO TODAY?

TOTAL STEPS:

STEP GOAL:

TOTAL CALORIES CONSUMED:

TOTAL CALORIES BURNED:

TOTAL FAT CONSUMED:

TOTAL FAT BURNED:

Daily Weight Loss Planner

Date: | Calorie limit: ____ kcal | fat limit: ____ g

TO DO LIST:

TODAY'S WEIGHT:

TODAY'S WORKOUT WILL INCLUDE:

TYPE: DURATION:

☐ CARDIO: ______________ ______________

☐ RESISTANCE: ______________ ______________

☐ CLASS/OTHER ______________ ______________

BREAKFAST

TIME:

CARB:

VEGGIE:

PROTEIN:

BEVERAGE:

SNACK: TIME:

TOTAL CALORIES AT THIS MEAL:

TOTAL FAT AT THIS MEAL:

LUNCH

TIME:

CARB:

VEGGIE:

PROTEIN:

BEVERAGE:

SNACK: TIME:

TOTAL CALORIES AT THIS MEAL:

TOTAL FAT AT THIS MEAL:

DINNER

TIME:

CARB:

VEGGIE:

PROTEIN:

BEVERAGE:

SNACK: TIME:

TOTAL CALORIES AT THIS MEAL:

TOTAL FAT AT THIS MEAL:

HOW DID I DO TODAY?

TOTAL STEPS:

STEP GOAL:

TOTAL CALORIES CONSUMED:

TOTAL CALORIES BURNED:

TOTAL FAT CONSUMED:

TOTAL FAT BURNED:

Daily Weight Loss Planner

Date: _______________   Calorie limit: _______ kcal | fat limit: _______ g

TO DO LIST:

TODAY'S WORKOUT WILL INCLUDE:

TYPE: DURATION:

☐ CARDIO: _____________ _____________

☐ RESISTANCE: _____________ _____________

TODAY'S WEIGHT:

☐ CLASS/OTHER _____________ _____________

BREAKFAST

TIME:

CARB:

VEGGIE:

PROTEIN:

BEVERAGE:

SNACK: TIME:

TOTAL CALORIES AT THIS MEAL:

TOTAL FAT AT THIS MEAL:

LUNCH

TIME:

CARB:

VEGGIE:

PROTEIN:

BEVERAGE:

SNACK: TIME:

TOTAL CALORIES AT THIS MEAL:

TOTAL FAT AT THIS MEAL:

DINNER

TIME:

CARB:

VEGGIE:

PROTEIN:

BEVERAGE:

SNACK: TIME:

TOTAL CALORIES AT THIS MEAL:

TOTAL FAT AT THIS MEAL:

HOW DID I DO TODAY?

TOTAL STEPS:

STEP GOAL:

TOTAL CALORIES CONSUMED:

TOTAL CALORIES BURNED:

TOTAL FAT CONSUMED:

TOTAL FAT BURNED:

Daily Weight Loss Planner

Date: ________________ Calorie limit: ______ kcal | fat limit: ______ g

TO DO LIST:

TODAY'S WORKOUT WILL INCLUDE:

	TYPE:	DURATION:
☐ CARDIO:	________________	________________
☐ RESISTANCE:	________________	________________
☐ CLASS/OTHER	________________	________________

TODAY'S WEIGHT:

BREAKFAST

TIME: ______ | TOTAL CALORIES AT THIS MEAL: | TOTAL FAT AT THIS MEAL:

CARB:

VEGGIE:

PROTEIN:

BEVERAGE:

SNACK: ______ TIME: ______

LUNCH

TIME: ______ | TOTAL CALORIES AT THIS MEAL: | TOTAL FAT AT THIS MEAL:

CARB:

VEGGIE:

PROTEIN:

BEVERAGE:

SNACK: ______ TIME: ______

DINNER

TIME: ______ | TOTAL CALORIES AT THIS MEAL: | TOTAL FAT AT THIS MEAL:

CARB:

VEGGIE:

PROTEIN:

BEVERAGE:

SNACK: ______ TIME: ______

HOW DID I DO TODAY?

TOTAL STEPS: ______ | TOTAL CALORIES CONSUMED: ______ | TOTAL FAT CONSUMED: ______

STEP GOAL: ______ | TOTAL CALORIES BURNED: ______ | TOTAL FAT BURNED: ______

Daily Weight Loss Planner

D a t e: Calorie limit: kcal | fat limit: g

TO DO LIST:

TODAY'S WEIGHT:

TODAY'S WORKOUT WILL INCLUDE:

TYPE: DURATION:

☐ CARDIO: ___________ ___________

☐ RESISTANCE: ___________ ___________

☐ CLASS/OTHER ___________ ___________

B R E A K F A S T

TIME:

CARB:

VEGGIE:

PROTEIN:

BEVERAGE:

SNACK: TIME:

TOTAL CALORIES AT THIS MEAL:

TOTAL FAT AT THIS MEAL:

L U N C H

TIME:

CARB:

VEGGIE:

PROTEIN:

BEVERAGE:

SNACK: TIME:

TOTAL CALORIES AT THIS MEAL:

TOTAL FAT AT THIS MEAL:

D I N N E R

TIME:

CARB:

VEGGIE:

PROTEIN:

BEVERAGE:

SNACK: TIME:

TOTAL CALORIES AT THIS MEAL:

TOTAL FAT AT THIS MEAL:

H O W   D I D   I   D O   TODAY?

TOTAL STEPS:

STEP GOAL:

TOTAL CALORIES CONSUMED:

TOTAL CALORIES BURNED:

TOTAL FAT CONSUMED:

TOTAL FAT BURNED:

Daily Weight Loss Planner

Date: Calorie limit: kcal | fat limit: g

TO DO LIST:

TODAY'S WORKOUT WILL INCLUDE:

TYPE: DURATION:

☐ CARDIO: _____________ _____________

☐ RESISTANCE: _____________ _____________

☐ CLASS/OTHER _____________ _____________

TODAY'S WEIGHT:

BREAKFAST
TIME:

CARB:

VEGGIE:

PROTEIN:

BEVERAGE:

SNACK: TIME:

TOTAL CALORIES AT THIS MEAL:	TOTAL FAT AT THIS MEAL:

LUNCH
TIME:

CARB:

VEGGIE:

PROTEIN:

BEVERAGE:

SNACK: TIME:

TOTAL CALORIES AT THIS MEAL:	TOTAL FAT AT THIS MEAL:

DINNER
TIME:

CARB:

VEGGIE:

PROTEIN:

BEVERAGE:

SNACK: TIME:

TOTAL CALORIES AT THIS MEAL:	TOTAL FAT AT THIS MEAL:

HOW DID I DO TODAY?

TOTAL STEPS:

STEP GOAL:

TOTAL CALORIES CONSUMED:	TOTAL FAT CONSUMED:
TOTAL CALORIES BURNED:	TOTAL FAT BURNED:

Daily Weight Loss Planner

Date: _______________   Calorie limit: _______ kcal | fat limit: _______ g

TO DO LIST:

TODAY'S WORKOUT WILL INCLUDE:

	TYPE:	DURATION:
☐ CARDIO:	_____________	_____________
☐ RESISTANCE:	_____________	_____________
☐ CLASS/OTHER	_____________	_____________

TODAY'S WEIGHT: _______________

B R E A K F A S T

TIME: _______________

- **CARB:**
- **VEGGIE:**
- **PROTEIN:**
- **BEVERAGE:**
- **SNACK:**   TIME: _______________

TOTAL CALORIES AT THIS MEAL:

TOTAL FAT AT THIS MEAL:

L U N C H

TIME: _______________

- **CARB:**
- **VEGGIE:**
- **PROTEIN:**
- **BEVERAGE:**
- **SNACK:**   TIME: _______________

TOTAL CALORIES AT THIS MEAL:

TOTAL FAT AT THIS MEAL:

D I N N E R

TIME: _______________

- **CARB:**
- **VEGGIE:**
- **PROTEIN:**
- **BEVERAGE:**
- **SNACK:**   TIME: _______________

TOTAL CALORIES AT THIS MEAL:

TOTAL FAT AT THIS MEAL:

H O W   D I D   I   D O   T O D A Y ?

TOTAL STEPS:

STEP GOAL:

TOTAL CALORIES CONSUMED:

TOTAL CALORIES BURNED:

TOTAL FAT CONSUMED:

TOTAL FAT BURNED:

Daily Weight Loss Planner

Date: Calorie limit: kcal | fat limit: g

TO DO LIST:

TODAY'S WORKOUT WILL INCLUDE:

	TYPE:	DURATION:
☐ CARDIO:	_____________	_____________
☐ RESISTANCE:	_____________	_____________
☐ CLASS/OTHER	_____________	_____________

TODAY'S WEIGHT:

BREAKFAST   TIME:

CARB:

VEGGIE:

PROTEIN:

BEVERAGE:

SNACK: TIME:

TOTAL CALORIES AT THIS MEAL:

TOTAL FAT AT THIS MEAL:

LUNCH   TIME:

CARB:

VEGGIE:

PROTEIN:

BEVERAGE:

SNACK: TIME:

TOTAL CALORIES AT THIS MEAL:

TOTAL FAT AT THIS MEAL:

DINNER   TIME:

CARB:

VEGGIE:

PROTEIN:

BEVERAGE:

SNACK: TIME:

TOTAL CALORIES AT THIS MEAL:

TOTAL FAT AT THIS MEAL:

HOW DID I DO TODAY?

TOTAL STEPS:

STEP GOAL:

TOTAL CALORIES CONSUMED:

TOTAL CALORIES BURNED:

TOTAL FAT CONSUMED:

TOTAL FAT BURNED:

Daily Weight Loss Planner

Date: ___________ Calorie limit: ___________ kcal | fat limit: ___________ g

TO DO LIST:

TODAY'S WEIGHT: ___________

TODAY'S WORKOUT WILL INCLUDE:

TYPE: DURATION:

☐ CARDIO: ___________ ___________

☐ RESISTANCE: ___________ ___________

☐ CLASS/OTHER ___________ ___________

BREAKFAST

TIME: ___________

CARB:

VEGGIE:

PROTEIN:

BEVERAGE:

SNACK: TIME: ___________

TOTAL CALORIES AT THIS MEAL:

TOTAL FAT AT THIS MEAL:

LUNCH

TIME: ___________

CARB:

VEGGIE:

PROTEIN:

BEVERAGE:

SNACK: TIME: ___________

TOTAL CALORIES AT THIS MEAL:

TOTAL FAT AT THIS MEAL:

DINNER

TIME: ___________

CARB:

VEGGIE:

PROTEIN:

BEVERAGE:

SNACK: TIME: ___________

TOTAL CALORIES AT THIS MEAL:

TOTAL FAT AT THIS MEAL:

HOW DID I DO TODAY?

TOTAL STEPS:

STEP GOAL:

TOTAL CALORIES CONSUMED:

TOTAL CALORIES BURNED:

TOTAL FAT CONSUMED:

TOTAL FAT BURNED:

Daily Weight Loss Planner

Date: ___________

Calorie limit: ______ kcal | fat limit: ______ g

TO DO LIST:

TODAY'S WORKOUT WILL INCLUDE:

TYPE: | DURATION:

☐ CARDIO: _______________ _______________

☐ RESISTANCE: _______________ _______________

☐ CLASS/OTHER _______________ _______________

TODAY'S WEIGHT:

BREAKFAST

TIME: ______

CARB:

VEGGIE:

PROTEIN:

BEVERAGE:

SNACK: ______ TIME: ______

TOTAL CALORIES AT THIS MEAL:

TOTAL FAT AT THIS MEAL:

LUNCH

TIME: ______

CARB:

VEGGIE:

PROTEIN:

BEVERAGE:

SNACK: ______ TIME: ______

TOTAL CALORIES AT THIS MEAL:

TOTAL FAT AT THIS MEAL:

DINNER

TIME: ______

CARB:

VEGGIE:

PROTEIN:

BEVERAGE:

SNACK: ______ TIME: ______

TOTAL CALORIES AT THIS MEAL:

TOTAL FAT AT THIS MEAL:

HOW DID I DO TODAY?

TOTAL STEPS:

STEP GOAL:

TOTAL CALORIES CONSUMED:

TOTAL CALORIES BURNED:

TOTAL FAT CONSUMED:

TOTAL FAT BURNED:

Daily Weight Loss Planner

D a t e :   Calorie limit: kcal | fat limit: g

TO DO LIST:

TODAY'S WORKOUT WILL INCLUDE:

TYPE: DURATION:

☐ CARDIO: ___________ ___________

☐ RESISTANCE: ___________ ___________

☐ CLASS/OTHER ___________ ___________

TODAY'S WEIGHT:

B R E A K F A S T

TIME:

TOTAL CALORIES AT THIS MEAL:

TOTAL FAT AT THIS MEAL:

CARB:

VEGGIE:

PROTEIN:

BEVERAGE:

SNACK: TIME:

L U N C H

TIME:

TOTAL CALORIES AT THIS MEAL:

TOTAL FAT AT THIS MEAL:

CARB:

VEGGIE:

PROTEIN:

BEVERAGE:

SNACK: TIME:

D I N N E R

TIME:

TOTAL CALORIES AT THIS MEAL:

TOTAL FAT AT THIS MEAL:

CARB:

VEGGIE:

PROTEIN:

BEVERAGE:

SNACK: TIME:

H O W   D I D   I   D O   T O D A Y ?

TOTAL STEPS:

TOTAL CALORIES CONSUMED:

TOTAL FAT CONSUMED:

STEP GOAL:

TOTAL CALORIES BURNED:

TOTAL FAT BURNED:

Daily Weight Loss Planner

Date: ___________________

Calorie limit: _______ kcal | fat limit: _______ g

TO DO LIST:

TODAY'S WEIGHT:

TODAY'S WORKOUT WILL INCLUDE:

	TYPE:	DURATION:
☐ CARDIO:	_____________	_____________
☐ RESISTANCE:	_____________	_____________
☐ CLASS/OTHER	_____________	_____________

BREAKFAST

TIME: _______

CARB:

VEGGIE:

PROTEIN:

BEVERAGE:

SNACK: TIME: _______

TOTAL CALORIES AT THIS MEAL:

TOTAL FAT AT THIS MEAL:

LUNCH

TIME: _______

CARB:

VEGGIE:

PROTEIN:

BEVERAGE:

SNACK: TIME: _______

TOTAL CALORIES AT THIS MEAL:

TOTAL FAT AT THIS MEAL:

DINNER

TIME: _______

CARB:

VEGGIE:

PROTEIN:

BEVERAGE:

SNACK: TIME: _______

TOTAL CALORIES AT THIS MEAL:

TOTAL FAT AT THIS MEAL:

HOW DID I DO TODAY?

TOTAL STEPS:

STEP GOAL:

TOTAL CALORIES CONSUMED:

TOTAL CALORIES BURNED:

TOTAL FAT CONSUMED:

TOTAL FAT BURNED:

Daily Weight Loss Planner

Date: **Calorie limit:**   kcal | **fat limit:**   g

TO DO LIST:

TODAY'S WORKOUT WILL INCLUDE:

TYPE: DURATION:

☐ CARDIO: _____________ _____________

☐ RESISTANCE: _____________ _____________

☐ CLASS/OTHER _____________ _____________

TODAY'S WEIGHT:

BREAKFAST

TIME:

CARB:

VEGGIE:

PROTEIN:

BEVERAGE:

SNACK: TIME:

TOTAL CALORIES AT THIS MEAL:

TOTAL FAT AT THIS MEAL:

LUNCH

TIME:

CARB:

VEGGIE:

PROTEIN:

BEVERAGE:

SNACK: TIME:

TOTAL CALORIES AT THIS MEAL:

TOTAL FAT AT THIS MEAL:

DINNER

TIME:

CARB:

VEGGIE:

PROTEIN:

BEVERAGE:

SNACK: TIME:

TOTAL CALORIES AT THIS MEAL:

TOTAL FAT AT THIS MEAL:

HOW DID I DO TODAY?

TOTAL STEPS:

STEP GOAL:

TOTAL CALORIES CONSUMED:

TOTAL CALORIES BURNED:

TOTAL FAT CONSUMED:

TOTAL FAT BURNED:

Daily Weight Loss Planner

Date: ___________________   Calorie limit: _______ kcal | fat limit: _______ g

TO DO LIST:

TODAY'S WORKOUT WILL INCLUDE:

TYPE: DURATION:

☐ CARDIO: _______________ _______________

☐ RESISTANCE: _______________ _______________

☐ CLASS/OTHER _______________ _______________

TODAY'S WEIGHT:

BREAKFAST

TIME:

CARB:

VEGGIE:

PROTEIN:

BEVERAGE:

SNACK: TIME:

TOTAL CALORIES AT THIS MEAL:

TOTAL FAT AT THIS MEAL:

LUNCH

TIME:

CARB:

VEGGIE:

PROTEIN:

BEVERAGE:

SNACK: TIME:

TOTAL CALORIES AT THIS MEAL:

TOTAL FAT AT THIS MEAL:

DINNER

TIME:

CARB:

VEGGIE:

PROTEIN:

BEVERAGE:

SNACK: TIME:

TOTAL CALORIES AT THIS MEAL:

TOTAL FAT AT THIS MEAL:

HOW DID I DO TODAY?

TOTAL STEPS:

STEP GOAL:

TOTAL CALORIES CONSUMED:

TOTAL CALORIES BURNED:

TOTAL FAT CONSUMED:

TOTAL FAT BURNED:

Daily Weight Loss Planner

D a t e: Calorie limit: kcal | fat limit: g

TO DO LIST:

TODAY'S WORKOUT WILL INCLUDE:

TYPE: DURATION:

☐ CARDIO: __________ __________

☐ RESISTANCE: __________ __________

☐ CLASS/OTHER __________ __________

TODAY'S WEIGHT:

B R E A K F A S T

TIME:

CARB:

VEGGIE:

PROTEIN:

BEVERAGE:

SNACK: TIME:

TOTAL CALORIES AT THIS MEAL:

TOTAL FAT AT THIS MEAL:

L U N C H

TIME:

CARB:

VEGGIE:

PROTEIN:

BEVERAGE:

SNACK: TIME:

TOTAL CALORIES AT THIS MEAL:

TOTAL FAT AT THIS MEAL:

D I N N E R

TIME:

CARB:

VEGGIE:

PROTEIN:

BEVERAGE:

SNACK: TIME:

TOTAL CALORIES AT THIS MEAL:

TOTAL FAT AT THIS MEAL:

H O W D I D I D O TODAY?

TOTAL STEPS:

STEP GOAL:

TOTAL CALORIES CONSUMED:

TOTAL CALORIES BURNED:

TOTAL FAT CONSUMED:

TOTAL FAT BURNED:

Daily Weight Loss Planner

Date: ________________   Calorie limit: ______ kcal | fat limit: ______ g

TO DO LIST:

TODAY'S WEIGHT:

TODAY'S WORKOUT WILL INCLUDE:

TYPE: DURATION:

☐ CARDIO: ________________ ________________

☐ RESISTANCE: ________________ ________________

☐ CLASS/OTHER ________________ ________________

BREAKFAST

CARB:

VEGGIE:

PROTEIN:

BEVERAGE:

SNACK:

TIME:

TIME:

TOTAL CALORIES AT THIS MEAL:

TOTAL FAT AT THIS MEAL:

LUNCH

CARB:

VEGGIE:

PROTEIN:

BEVERAGE:

SNACK:

TIME:

TIME:

TOTAL CALORIES AT THIS MEAL:

TOTAL FAT AT THIS MEAL:

DINNER

CARB:

VEGGIE:

PROTEIN:

BEVERAGE:

SNACK:

TIME:

TIME:

TOTAL CALORIES AT THIS MEAL:

TOTAL FAT AT THIS MEAL:

HOW DID I DO TODAY?

TOTAL STEPS:

STEP GOAL:

TOTAL CALORIES CONSUMED:

TOTAL CALORIES BURNED:

TOTAL FAT CONSUMED:

TOTAL FAT BURNED:

Daily Weight Loss Planner

Date: **Calorie limit:**   kcal | **fat limit:**   g

TO DO LIST:

TODAY'S WORKOUT WILL INCLUDE:

	TYPE:	DURATION:
☐ CARDIO:	_____________	_____________
☐ RESISTANCE:	_____________	_____________
☐ CLASS/OTHER	_____________	_____________

TODAY'S WEIGHT:

BREAKFAST

TIME:

CARB:

VEGGIE:

PROTEIN:

BEVERAGE:

SNACK: TIME:

TOTAL CALORIES AT THIS MEAL:

TOTAL FAT AT THIS MEAL:

LUNCH

TIME:

CARB:

VEGGIE:

PROTEIN:

BEVERAGE:

SNACK: TIME:

TOTAL CALORIES AT THIS MEAL:

TOTAL FAT AT THIS MEAL:

DINNER

TIME:

CARB:

VEGGIE:

PROTEIN:

BEVERAGE:

SNACK: TIME:

TOTAL CALORIES AT THIS MEAL:

TOTAL FAT AT THIS MEAL:

HOW DID I DO TODAY?

TOTAL STEPS:

STEP GOAL:

TOTAL CALORIES CONSUMED:

TOTAL CALORIES BURNED:

TOTAL FAT CONSUMED:

TOTAL FAT BURNED:

Daily Weight Loss Planner

Date: ____________________ Calorie limit: ______ kcal | fat limit: ______ g

TO DO LIST:

TODAY'S WEIGHT:

TODAY'S WORKOUT WILL INCLUDE:

TYPE: DURATION:

☐ CARDIO: ____________ ____________

☐ RESISTANCE: ____________ ____________

☐ CLASS/OTHER ____________ ____________

B R E A K F A S T

TIME:

CARB:

VEGGIE:

PROTEIN:

BEVERAGE:

SNACK: TIME:

TOTAL CALORIES AT THIS MEAL:

TOTAL FAT AT THIS MEAL:

L U N C H

TIME:

CARB:

VEGGIE:

PROTEIN:

BEVERAGE:

SNACK: TIME:

TOTAL CALORIES AT THIS MEAL:

TOTAL FAT AT THIS MEAL:

D I N N E R

TIME:

CARB:

VEGGIE:

PROTEIN:

BEVERAGE:

SNACK: TIME:

TOTAL CALORIES AT THIS MEAL:

TOTAL FAT AT THIS MEAL:

H O W   D I D   I   D O   TODAY?

TOTAL STEPS:

STEP GOAL:

TOTAL CALORIES CONSUMED:

TOTAL CALORIES BURNED:

TOTAL FAT CONSUMED:

TOTAL FAT BURNED:

Daily Weight Loss Planner

Date: ___________   Calorie limit: ______ kcal | fat limit: ______ g

TO DO LIST:

TODAY'S WEIGHT: ___________

TODAY'S WORKOUT WILL INCLUDE:

		TYPE:	DURATION:
☐	CARDIO:	_________	_________
☐	RESISTANCE:	_________	_________
☐	CLASS/OTHER	_________	_________

BREAKFAST

TIME: ___________

CARB:

VEGGIE:

PROTEIN:

BEVERAGE:

SNACK: ___________ TIME: ___________

TOTAL CALORIES AT THIS MEAL:

TOTAL FAT AT THIS MEAL:

LUNCH

TIME: ___________

CARB:

VEGGIE:

PROTEIN:

BEVERAGE:

SNACK: ___________ TIME: ___________

TOTAL CALORIES AT THIS MEAL:

TOTAL FAT AT THIS MEAL:

DINNER

TIME: ___________

CARB:

VEGGIE:

PROTEIN:

BEVERAGE:

SNACK: ___________ TIME: ___________

TOTAL CALORIES AT THIS MEAL:

TOTAL FAT AT THIS MEAL:

HOW DID I DO TODAY?

TOTAL STEPS:

STEP GOAL:

TOTAL CALORIES CONSUMED:

TOTAL CALORIES BURNED:

TOTAL FAT CONSUMED:

TOTAL FAT BURNED:

Daily Weight Loss Planner

Date: Calorie limit: kcal | fat limit: g

TO DO LIST:

TODAY'S WORKOUT WILL INCLUDE:

	TYPE:	DURATION:
☐ CARDIO:	_____________	_____________
☐ RESISTANCE:	_____________	_____________
☐ CLASS/OTHER	_____________	_____________

TODAY'S WEIGHT:

BREAKFAST

TIME:

CARB:

VEGGIE:

PROTEIN:

BEVERAGE:

SNACK: TIME:

TOTAL CALORIES AT THIS MEAL:

TOTAL FAT AT THIS MEAL:

LUNCH

TIME:

CARB:

VEGGIE:

PROTEIN:

BEVERAGE:

SNACK: TIME:

TOTAL CALORIES AT THIS MEAL:

TOTAL FAT AT THIS MEAL:

DINNER

TIME:

CARB:

VEGGIE:

PROTEIN:

BEVERAGE:

SNACK: TIME:

TOTAL CALORIES AT THIS MEAL:

TOTAL FAT AT THIS MEAL:

HOW DID I DO TODAY?

TOTAL STEPS:

STEP GOAL:

TOTAL CALORIES CONSUMED:

TOTAL CALORIES BURNED:

TOTAL FAT CONSUMED:

TOTAL FAT BURNED:

Daily Weight Loss Planner

D a t e :   Calorie limit: kcal | fat limit: g

TO DO LIST:

TODAY'S WORKOUT WILL INCLUDE:

TYPE: DURATION:

☐ CARDIO: ____________ ____________

☐ RESISTANCE: ____________ ____________

☐ CLASS/OTHER ____________ ____________

TODAY'S WEIGHT:

B R E A K F A S T

TIME: TOTAL CALORIES AT THIS MEAL: TOTAL FAT AT THIS MEAL:

CARB:

VEGGIE:

PROTEIN:

BEVERAGE:

SNACK: TIME:

L U N C H

TIME: TOTAL CALORIES AT THIS MEAL: TOTAL FAT AT THIS MEAL:

CARB:

VEGGIE:

PROTEIN:

BEVERAGE:

SNACK: TIME:

D I N N E R

TIME: TOTAL CALORIES AT THIS MEAL: TOTAL FAT AT THIS MEAL:

CARB:

VEGGIE:

PROTEIN:

BEVERAGE:

SNACK: TIME:

H O W   D I D   I   D O   T O D A Y ?

TOTAL STEPS: TOTAL CALORIES CONSUMED: TOTAL FAT CONSUMED:

STEP GOAL: TOTAL CALORIES BURNED: TOTAL FAT BURNED:

Daily Weight Loss Planner

Date: | Calorie limit: ___ kcal | fat limit: ___ g

TO DO LIST:

TODAY'S WEIGHT:

TODAY'S WORKOUT WILL INCLUDE:

	TYPE:	DURATION:
☐ CARDIO:	_______________	_______________
☐ RESISTANCE:	_______________	_______________
☐ CLASS/OTHER	_______________	_______________

BREAKFAST

TIME:

CARB:

VEGGIE:

PROTEIN:

BEVERAGE:

SNACK: TIME:

TOTAL CALORIES AT THIS MEAL:

TOTAL FAT AT THIS MEAL:

LUNCH

TIME:

CARB:

VEGGIE:

PROTEIN:

BEVERAGE:

SNACK: TIME:

TOTAL CALORIES AT THIS MEAL:

TOTAL FAT AT THIS MEAL:

DINNER

TIME:

CARB:

VEGGIE:

PROTEIN:

BEVERAGE:

SNACK: TIME:

TOTAL CALORIES AT THIS MEAL:

TOTAL FAT AT THIS MEAL:

HOW DID I DO TODAY?

TOTAL STEPS:

STEP GOAL:

TOTAL CALORIES CONSUMED:

TOTAL CALORIES BURNED:

TOTAL FAT CONSUMED:

TOTAL FAT BURNED:

Daily Weight Loss Planner

Date: _______________   Calorie limit: _______ kcal | fat limit: _____ g

TO DO LIST:

TODAY'S WEIGHT:

TODAY'S WORKOUT WILL INCLUDE:

TYPE: DURATION:

☐ CARDIO: _____________ _____________

☐ RESISTANCE: _____________ _____________

☐ CLASS/OTHER _____________ _____________

BREAKFAST

TIME:

CARB:

VEGGIE:

PROTEIN:

BEVERAGE:

SNACK: TIME:

TOTAL CALORIES AT THIS MEAL:

TOTAL FAT AT THIS MEAL:

LUNCH

TIME:

CARB:

VEGGIE:

PROTEIN:

BEVERAGE:

SNACK: TIME:

TOTAL CALORIES AT THIS MEAL:

TOTAL FAT AT THIS MEAL:

DINNER

TIME:

CARB:

VEGGIE:

PROTEIN:

BEVERAGE:

SNACK: TIME:

TOTAL CALORIES AT THIS MEAL:

TOTAL FAT AT THIS MEAL:

HOW DID I DO TODAY?

TOTAL STEPS:

STEP GOAL:

TOTAL CALORIES CONSUMED:

TOTAL CALORIES BURNED:

TOTAL FAT CONSUMED:

TOTAL FAT BURNED:

Daily Weight Loss Planner

Date: ___________   Calorie limit: ________ kcal | fat limit: ____ g

TO DO LIST:

TODAY'S WORKOUT WILL INCLUDE:

	TYPE:	DURATION:
☐ CARDIO:	___________	___________
☐ RESISTANCE:	___________	___________
☐ CLASS/OTHER	___________	___________

TODAY'S WEIGHT:

BREAKFAST

TIME: ___________   TOTAL CALORIES AT THIS MEAL: ___________   TOTAL FAT AT THIS MEAL: ___________

CARB:

VEGGIE:

PROTEIN:

BEVERAGE:

SNACK: TIME:

LUNCH

TIME: ___________   TOTAL CALORIES AT THIS MEAL: ___________   TOTAL FAT AT THIS MEAL: ___________

CARB:

VEGGIE:

PROTEIN:

BEVERAGE:

SNACK: TIME:

DINNER

TIME: ___________   TOTAL CALORIES AT THIS MEAL: ___________   TOTAL FAT AT THIS MEAL: ___________

CARB:

VEGGIE:

PROTEIN:

BEVERAGE:

SNACK: TIME:

HOW DID I DO TODAY?

TOTAL STEPS: ___________   TOTAL CALORIES CONSUMED: ___________   TOTAL FAT CONSUMED: ___________

STEP GOAL: ___________   TOTAL CALORIES BURNED: ___________   TOTAL FAT BURNED: ___________

Daily Weight Loss Planner

Date: Calorie limit: kcal | fat limit: g

TO DO LIST:

TODAY'S WORKOUT WILL INCLUDE:

               TYPE: DURATION:

☐ CARDIO: ___________ ___________

☐ RESISTANCE: ___________ ___________

☐ CLASS/OTHER ___________ ___________

TODAY'S WEIGHT:

BREAKFAST

TIME:

CARB:

VEGGIE:

PROTEIN:

BEVERAGE:

SNACK: TIME:

TOTAL CALORIES AT THIS MEAL:	TOTAL FAT AT THIS MEAL:

LUNCH

TIME:

CARB:

VEGGIE:

PROTEIN:

BEVERAGE:

SNACK: TIME:

TOTAL CALORIES AT THIS MEAL:	TOTAL FAT AT THIS MEAL:

DINNER

TIME:

CARB:

VEGGIE:

PROTEIN:

BEVERAGE:

SNACK: TIME:

TOTAL CALORIES AT THIS MEAL:	TOTAL FAT AT THIS MEAL:

HOW DID I DO TODAY?

	TOTAL CALORIES CONSUMED:	TOTAL FAT CONSUMED:
TOTAL STEPS:		
STEP GOAL:	TOTAL CALORIES BURNED:	TOTAL FAT BURNED:

Daily Weight Loss Planner

Date:

Calorie limit: _____ kcal | fat limit: _____ g

TO DO LIST:

TODAY'S WEIGHT:

TODAY'S WORKOUT WILL INCLUDE:

TYPE: DURATION:

☐ **CARDIO:** _____________ _____________

☐ **RESISTANCE:** _____________ _____________

☐ **CLASS/OTHER** _____________ _____________

BREAKFAST

TIME:

CARB:

VEGGIE:

PROTEIN:

BEVERAGE:

SNACK: TIME:

TOTAL CALORIES AT THIS MEAL:

TOTAL FAT AT THIS MEAL:

LUNCH

TIME:

CARB:

VEGGIE:

PROTEIN:

BEVERAGE:

SNACK: TIME:

TOTAL CALORIES AT THIS MEAL:

TOTAL FAT AT THIS MEAL:

DINNER

TIME:

CARB:

VEGGIE:

PROTEIN:

BEVERAGE:

SNACK: TIME:

TOTAL CALORIES AT THIS MEAL:

TOTAL FAT AT THIS MEAL:

HOW DID I DO TODAY?

TOTAL STEPS:

STEP GOAL:

TOTAL CALORIES CONSUMED:

TOTAL CALORIES BURNED:

TOTAL FAT CONSUMED:

TOTAL FAT BURNED:

Daily Weight Loss Planner

Date: _______________ Calorie limit: _______ kcal | fat limit: _______ g

TO DO LIST:

TODAY'S WEIGHT: _______

TODAY'S WORKOUT WILL INCLUDE:

	TYPE:	DURATION:
☐ CARDIO:	_____________	_____________
☐ RESISTANCE:	_____________	_____________
☐ CLASS/OTHER	_____________	_____________

BREAKFAST

TIME: _______ TOTAL CALORIES AT THIS MEAL: _______ TOTAL FAT AT THIS MEAL: _______

CARB:

VEGGIE:

PROTEIN:

BEVERAGE:

SNACK: TIME: _______

LUNCH

TIME: _______ TOTAL CALORIES AT THIS MEAL: _______ TOTAL FAT AT THIS MEAL: _______

CARB:

VEGGIE:

PROTEIN:

BEVERAGE:

SNACK: TIME: _______

DINNER

TIME: _______ TOTAL CALORIES AT THIS MEAL: _______ TOTAL FAT AT THIS MEAL: _______

CARB:

VEGGIE:

PROTEIN:

BEVERAGE:

SNACK: TIME: _______

HOW DID I DO TODAY?

TOTAL STEPS: _______ TOTAL CALORIES CONSUMED: _______ TOTAL FAT CONSUMED: _______

STEP GOAL: _______ TOTAL CALORIES BURNED: _______ TOTAL FAT BURNED: _______

Daily Weight Loss Planner

Date: ____________________   Calorie limit: ______ kcal | fat limit: ______ g

TO DO LIST:

TODAY'S WORKOUT WILL INCLUDE:

	TYPE:	DURATION:
☐ CARDIO:	______________	______________
☐ RESISTANCE:	______________	______________
☐ CLASS/OTHER	______________	______________

TODAY'S WEIGHT:

BREAKFAST   TIME:

	TOTAL CALORIES AT THIS MEAL:	TOTAL FAT AT THIS MEAL:

CARB:

VEGGIE:

PROTEIN:

BEVERAGE:

SNACK: TIME:

LUNCH   TIME:

	TOTAL CALORIES AT THIS MEAL:	TOTAL FAT AT THIS MEAL:

CARB:

VEGGIE:

PROTEIN:

BEVERAGE:

SNACK: TIME:

DINNER   TIME:

	TOTAL CALORIES AT THIS MEAL:	TOTAL FAT AT THIS MEAL:

CARB:

VEGGIE:

PROTEIN:

BEVERAGE:

SNACK: TIME:

HOW DID I DO TODAY?

	TOTAL CALORIES CONSUMED:	TOTAL FAT CONSUMED:
TOTAL STEPS:		
STEP GOAL:	TOTAL CALORIES BURNED:	TOTAL FAT BURNED:

Daily Weight Loss Planner

Date: Calorie limit: kcal | fat limit: g

TO DO LIST:

TODAY'S WORKOUT WILL INCLUDE:

TYPE: DURATION:

☐ CARDIO: _____________ _____________

☐ RESISTANCE: _____________ _____________

☐ CLASS/OTHER _____________ _____________

TODAY'S WEIGHT:

BREAKFAST

TIME:

TOTAL CALORIES AT THIS MEAL:

TOTAL FAT AT THIS MEAL:

CARB:

VEGGIE:

PROTEIN:

BEVERAGE:

SNACK: TIME:

LUNCH

TIME:

TOTAL CALORIES AT THIS MEAL:

TOTAL FAT AT THIS MEAL:

CARB:

VEGGIE:

PROTEIN:

BEVERAGE:

SNACK: TIME:

DINNER

TIME:

TOTAL CALORIES AT THIS MEAL:

TOTAL FAT AT THIS MEAL:

CARB:

VEGGIE:

PROTEIN:

BEVERAGE:

SNACK: TIME:

HOW DID I DO TODAY?

TOTAL STEPS:

STEP GOAL:

TOTAL CALORIES CONSUMED:

TOTAL CALORIES BURNED:

TOTAL FAT CONSUMED:

TOTAL FAT BURNED:

Daily Weight Loss Planner

Date: Calorie limit: ____ kcal | fat limit: ____ g

TO DO LIST:

TODAY'S WORKOUT WILL INCLUDE:

TYPE: DURATION:

☐ CARDIO: ____________ ____________

☐ RESISTANCE: ____________ ____________

☐ CLASS/OTHER ____________ ____________

TODAY'S WEIGHT:

BREAKFAST

TIME:

CARB:

VEGGIE:

PROTEIN:

BEVERAGE:

SNACK: TIME:

TOTAL CALORIES AT THIS MEAL:

TOTAL FAT AT THIS MEAL:

LUNCH

TIME:

CARB:

VEGGIE:

PROTEIN:

BEVERAGE:

SNACK: TIME:

TOTAL CALORIES AT THIS MEAL:

TOTAL FAT AT THIS MEAL:

DINNER

TIME:

CARB:

VEGGIE:

PROTEIN:

BEVERAGE:

SNACK: TIME:

TOTAL CALORIES AT THIS MEAL:

TOTAL FAT AT THIS MEAL:

HOW DID I DO TODAY?

TOTAL STEPS:

STEP GOAL:

TOTAL CALORIES CONSUMED:

TOTAL CALORIES BURNED:

TOTAL FAT CONSUMED:

TOTAL FAT BURNED:

Daily Weight Loss Planner

Date: _______________   Calorie limit: _______ kcal | fat limit: _______ g

TO DO LIST:

TODAY'S WORKOUT WILL INCLUDE:

TYPE: DURATION:

☐ CARDIO: _____________ _____________

☐ RESISTANCE: _____________ _____________

☐ CLASS/OTHER _____________ _____________

TODAY'S WEIGHT:

B R E A K F A S T   TIME: _______

CARB:

VEGGIE:

PROTEIN:

BEVERAGE:

SNACK: TIME: _______

TOTAL CALORIES AT THIS MEAL:

TOTAL FAT AT THIS MEAL:

L U N C H   TIME: _______

CARB:

VEGGIE:

PROTEIN:

BEVERAGE:

SNACK: TIME: _______

TOTAL CALORIES AT THIS MEAL:

TOTAL FAT AT THIS MEAL:

D I N N E R   TIME: _______

CARB:

VEGGIE:

PROTEIN:

BEVERAGE:

SNACK: TIME: _______

TOTAL CALORIES AT THIS MEAL:

TOTAL FAT AT THIS MEAL:

H O W   D I D   I   D O   T O D A Y ?

TOTAL STEPS:

STEP GOAL:

TOTAL CALORIES CONSUMED:

TOTAL CALORIES BURNED:

TOTAL FAT CONSUMED:

TOTAL FAT BURNED:

Daily Weight Loss Planner

Date:

Calorie limit: ______ kcal | fat limit: ______ g

TO DO LIST:

TODAY'S WEIGHT:

TODAY'S WORKOUT WILL INCLUDE:

	TYPE:	DURATION:
☐ CARDIO:	__________	__________
☐ RESISTANCE:	__________	__________
☐ CLASS/OTHER	__________	__________

BREAKFAST

TIME:

CARB:

VEGGIE:

PROTEIN:

BEVERAGE:

SNACK: TIME:

TOTAL CALORIES AT THIS MEAL:

TOTAL FAT AT THIS MEAL:

LUNCH

TIME:

CARB:

VEGGIE:

PROTEIN:

BEVERAGE:

SNACK: TIME:

TOTAL CALORIES AT THIS MEAL:

TOTAL FAT AT THIS MEAL:

DINNER

TIME:

CARB:

VEGGIE:

PROTEIN:

BEVERAGE:

SNACK: TIME:

TOTAL CALORIES AT THIS MEAL:

TOTAL FAT AT THIS MEAL:

HOW DID I DO TODAY?

TOTAL STEPS:

STEP GOAL:

TOTAL CALORIES CONSUMED:

TOTAL CALORIES BURNED:

TOTAL FAT CONSUMED:

TOTAL FAT BURNED:

Daily Weight Loss Planner

Date: Calorie limit: kcal | fat limit: g

TO DO LIST:

TODAY'S WEIGHT:

TODAY'S WORKOUT WILL INCLUDE:

	TYPE:	DURATION:
☐ CARDIO:	_____________	_____________
☐ RESISTANCE:	_____________	_____________
☐ CLASS/OTHER	_____________	_____________

BREAKFAST

TIME:

CARB:

VEGGIE:

PROTEIN:

BEVERAGE:

SNACK: TIME:

TOTAL CALORIES AT THIS MEAL:

TOTAL FAT AT THIS MEAL:

LUNCH

TIME:

CARB:

VEGGIE:

PROTEIN:

BEVERAGE:

SNACK: TIME:

TOTAL CALORIES AT THIS MEAL:

TOTAL FAT AT THIS MEAL:

DINNER

TIME:

CARB:

VEGGIE:

PROTEIN:

BEVERAGE:

SNACK: TIME:

TOTAL CALORIES AT THIS MEAL:

TOTAL FAT AT THIS MEAL:

HOW DID I DO TODAY?

TOTAL STEPS:

STEP GOAL:

TOTAL CALORIES CONSUMED:

TOTAL CALORIES BURNED:

TOTAL FAT CONSUMED:

TOTAL FAT BURNED:

Daily Weight Loss Planner

Date: Calorie limit: kcal | fat limit: g

TO DO LIST:

TODAY'S WORKOUT WILL INCLUDE:

TYPE: DURATION:

☐ CARDIO: ____________ ____________

☐ RESISTANCE: ____________ ____________

☐ CLASS/OTHER ____________ ____________

TODAY'S WEIGHT:

B R E A K F A S T

TIME:

CARB:

VEGGIE:

PROTEIN:

BEVERAGE:

SNACK: TIME:

TOTAL CALORIES AT THIS MEAL:

TOTAL FAT AT THIS MEAL:

L U N C H

TIME:

CARB:

VEGGIE:

PROTEIN:

BEVERAGE:

SNACK: TIME:

TOTAL CALORIES AT THIS MEAL:

TOTAL FAT AT THIS MEAL:

D I N N E R

TIME:

CARB:

VEGGIE:

PROTEIN:

BEVERAGE:

SNACK: TIME:

TOTAL CALORIES AT THIS MEAL:

TOTAL FAT AT THIS MEAL:

H O W   D I D   I   D O   T O D A Y ?

TOTAL STEPS:

STEP GOAL:

TOTAL CALORIES CONSUMED:

TOTAL CALORIES BURNED:

TOTAL FAT CONSUMED:

TOTAL FAT BURNED:

Daily Weight Loss Planner

Date: _______________   Calorie limit: _______ kcal | fat limit: _______ g

TO DO LIST:

TODAY'S WORKOUT WILL INCLUDE:

	TYPE:	DURATION:
☐ CARDIO:	_____________	_____________
☐ RESISTANCE:	_____________	_____________
☐ CLASS/OTHER	_____________	_____________

TODAY'S WEIGHT:

BREAKFAST   TIME: _______

TOTAL CALORIES AT THIS MEAL: _______   TOTAL FAT AT THIS MEAL: _______

- **CARB:**
- **VEGGIE:**
- **PROTEIN:**
- **BEVERAGE:**
- **SNACK:**   TIME: _______

LUNCH   TIME: _______

TOTAL CALORIES AT THIS MEAL: _______   TOTAL FAT AT THIS MEAL: _______

- **CARB:**
- **VEGGIE:**
- **PROTEIN:**
- **BEVERAGE:**
- **SNACK:**   TIME: _______

DINNER   TIME: _______

TOTAL CALORIES AT THIS MEAL: _______   TOTAL FAT AT THIS MEAL: _______

- **CARB:**
- **VEGGIE:**
- **PROTEIN:**
- **BEVERAGE:**
- **SNACK:**   TIME: _______

HOW DID I DO TODAY?

TOTAL STEPS:	TOTAL CALORIES CONSUMED:	TOTAL FAT CONSUMED:
STEP GOAL:	TOTAL CALORIES BURNED:	TOTAL FAT BURNED:

Daily Weight Loss Planner

Date: | Calorie limit: kcal | fat limit: g

TO DO LIST:

TODAY'S WORKOUT WILL INCLUDE:

TYPE: DURATION:

☐ CARDIO: ______________   ______________

☐ RESISTANCE: ______________   ______________

☐ CLASS/OTHER   ______________   ______________

TODAY'S WEIGHT:

BREAKFAST

TIME:

TOTAL CALORIES AT THIS MEAL:

TOTAL FAT AT THIS MEAL:

CARB:

VEGGIE:

PROTEIN:

BEVERAGE:

SNACK: TIME:

LUNCH

TIME:

TOTAL CALORIES AT THIS MEAL:

TOTAL FAT AT THIS MEAL:

CARB:

VEGGIE:

PROTEIN:

BEVERAGE:

SNACK: TIME:

DINNER

TIME:

TOTAL CALORIES AT THIS MEAL:

TOTAL FAT AT THIS MEAL:

CARB:

VEGGIE:

PROTEIN:

BEVERAGE:

SNACK: TIME:

HOW DID I DO TODAY?

TOTAL STEPS:

STEP GOAL:

TOTAL CALORIES CONSUMED:

TOTAL CALORIES BURNED:

TOTAL FAT CONSUMED:

TOTAL FAT BURNED:

Daily Weight Loss Planner

D a t e : Calorie limit: kcal | fat limit: g

TO DO LIST:

TODAY'S WORKOUT WILL INCLUDE:

TYPE: DURATION:

☐ CARDIO: ___________ ___________

☐ RESISTANCE: ___________ ___________

TODAY'S WEIGHT:

☐ CLASS/OTHER ___________ ___________

B R E A K F A S T

TIME:

CARB:

VEGGIE:

PROTEIN:

BEVERAGE:

SNACK: TIME:

TOTAL CALORIES AT THIS MEAL:

TOTAL FAT AT THIS MEAL:

L U N C H

TIME:

CARB:

VEGGIE:

PROTEIN:

BEVERAGE:

SNACK: TIME:

TOTAL CALORIES AT THIS MEAL:

TOTAL FAT AT THIS MEAL:

D I N N E R

TIME:

CARB:

VEGGIE:

PROTEIN:

BEVERAGE:

SNACK: TIME:

TOTAL CALORIES AT THIS MEAL:

TOTAL FAT AT THIS MEAL:

H O W   D I D   I   D O   T O D A Y ?

TOTAL STEPS:

STEP GOAL:

TOTAL CALORIES CONSUMED:

TOTAL CALORIES BURNED:

TOTAL FAT CONSUMED:

TOTAL FAT BURNED:

Daily Weight Loss Planner

Date: Calorie limit: ______ kcal | fat limit: ______ g

TO DO LIST:

TODAY'S WEIGHT:

TODAY'S WORKOUT WILL INCLUDE:

TYPE: DURATION:

☐ CARDIO: ______________ ______________

☐ RESISTANCE: ______________ ______________

☐ CLASS/OTHER ______________ ______________

BREAKFAST

TIME:

CARB:

VEGGIE:

PROTEIN:

BEVERAGE:

SNACK: TIME:

TOTAL CALORIES AT THIS MEAL:

TOTAL FAT AT THIS MEAL:

LUNCH

TIME:

CARB:

VEGGIE:

PROTEIN:

BEVERAGE:

SNACK: TIME:

TOTAL CALORIES AT THIS MEAL:

TOTAL FAT AT THIS MEAL:

DINNER

TIME:

CARB:

VEGGIE:

PROTEIN:

BEVERAGE:

SNACK: TIME:

TOTAL CALORIES AT THIS MEAL:

TOTAL FAT AT THIS MEAL:

HOW DID I DO TODAY?

TOTAL STEPS:

STEP GOAL:

TOTAL CALORIES CONSUMED:

TOTAL CALORIES BURNED:

TOTAL FAT CONSUMED:

TOTAL FAT BURNED:

Daily Weight Loss Planner

Date: Calorie limit: kcal | fat limit: g

TO DO LIST:

TODAY'S WEIGHT:

TODAY'S WORKOUT WILL INCLUDE:

	TYPE:	DURATION:
☐ CARDIO:	____________	____________
☐ RESISTANCE:	____________	____________
☐ CLASS/OTHER	____________	____________

BREAKFAST

TIME:

- CARB:
- VEGGIE:
- PROTEIN:
- BEVERAGE:
- SNACK: TIME:

TOTAL CALORIES AT THIS MEAL:

TOTAL FAT AT THIS MEAL:

LUNCH

TIME:

- CARB:
- VEGGIE:
- PROTEIN:
- BEVERAGE:
- SNACK: TIME:

TOTAL CALORIES AT THIS MEAL:

TOTAL FAT AT THIS MEAL:

DINNER

TIME:

- CARB:
- VEGGIE:
- PROTEIN:
- BEVERAGE:
- SNACK: TIME:

TOTAL CALORIES AT THIS MEAL:

TOTAL FAT AT THIS MEAL:

HOW DID I DO TODAY?

TOTAL STEPS:

STEP GOAL:

TOTAL CALORIES CONSUMED:

TOTAL CALORIES BURNED:

TOTAL FAT CONSUMED:

TOTAL FAT BURNED:

Daily Weight Loss Planner

Date: ___________

Calorie limit: _______ kcal | fat limit: _______ g

TO DO LIST:

TODAY'S WORKOUT WILL INCLUDE:

TYPE: DURATION:

☐ CARDIO: _____________ _____________

☐ RESISTANCE: _____________ _____________

☐ CLASS/OTHER _____________ _____________

TODAY'S WEIGHT:

BREAKFAST   TIME: _______

CARB:

VEGGIE:

PROTEIN:

BEVERAGE:

SNACK: _______   TIME: _______

TOTAL CALORIES AT THIS MEAL:	TOTAL FAT AT THIS MEAL:

LUNCH   TIME: _______

CARB:

VEGGIE:

PROTEIN:

BEVERAGE:

SNACK: _______   TIME: _______

TOTAL CALORIES AT THIS MEAL:	TOTAL FAT AT THIS MEAL:

DINNER   TIME: _______

CARB:

VEGGIE:

PROTEIN:

BEVERAGE:

SNACK: _______   TIME: _______

TOTAL CALORIES AT THIS MEAL:	TOTAL FAT AT THIS MEAL:

HOW DID I DO TODAY?

TOTAL STEPS:

STEP GOAL:

TOTAL CALORIES CONSUMED:

TOTAL CALORIES BURNED:

TOTAL FAT CONSUMED:

TOTAL FAT BURNED:

Daily Weight Loss Planner

D a t e :   Calorie limit: kcal | fat limit: g

TO DO LIST:

TODAY'S WORKOUT WILL INCLUDE:

TYPE: DURATION:

☐ CARDIO: _______________ _______________

☐ RESISTANCE: _______________ _______________

☐ CLASS/OTHER _______________ _______________

TODAY'S WEIGHT:

B R E A K F A S T

TIME:

CARB:

VEGGIE:

PROTEIN:

BEVERAGE:

SNACK: TIME:

TOTAL CALORIES AT THIS MEAL:

TOTAL FAT AT THIS MEAL:

L U N C H

TIME:

CARB:

VEGGIE:

PROTEIN:

BEVERAGE:

SNACK: TIME:

TOTAL CALORIES AT THIS MEAL:

TOTAL FAT AT THIS MEAL:

D I N N E R

TIME:

CARB:

VEGGIE:

PROTEIN:

BEVERAGE:

SNACK: TIME:

TOTAL CALORIES AT THIS MEAL:

TOTAL FAT AT THIS MEAL:

H O W D I D I D O T O D A Y ?

TOTAL STEPS:

STEP GOAL:

TOTAL CALORIES CONSUMED:

TOTAL CALORIES BURNED:

TOTAL FAT CONSUMED:

TOTAL FAT BURNED:

Daily Weight Loss Planner

Date: ______________   Calorie limit: ______ kcal | fat limit: ______ g

TO DO LIST:

TODAY'S WORKOUT WILL INCLUDE:

		TYPE:	DURATION:
☐	CARDIO:	_____________	_____________
☐	RESISTANCE:	_____________	_____________
☐	CLASS/OTHER	_____________	_____________

TODAY'S WEIGHT:

BREAKFAST   TIME:

CARB:

VEGGIE:

PROTEIN:

BEVERAGE:

SNACK: TIME:

TOTAL CALORIES AT THIS MEAL:

TOTAL FAT AT THIS MEAL:

LUNCH   TIME:

CARB:

VEGGIE:

PROTEIN:

BEVERAGE:

SNACK: TIME:

TOTAL CALORIES AT THIS MEAL:

TOTAL FAT AT THIS MEAL:

DINNER   TIME:

CARB:

VEGGIE:

PROTEIN:

BEVERAGE:

SNACK: TIME:

TOTAL CALORIES AT THIS MEAL:

TOTAL FAT AT THIS MEAL:

HOW DID I DO TODAY?

TOTAL STEPS:

STEP GOAL:

TOTAL CALORIES CONSUMED:

TOTAL CALORIES BURNED:

TOTAL FAT CONSUMED:

TOTAL FAT BURNED:

Daily Weight Loss Planner

Date: ____________   Calorie limit: ________ kcal | fat limit: ____ g

TO DO LIST:

TODAY'S WORKOUT WILL INCLUDE:

TYPE: DURATION:

☐ CARDIO: ____________ ____________

☐ RESISTANCE: ____________ ____________

☐ CLASS/OTHER ____________ ____________

TODAY'S WEIGHT: ____________

BREAKFAST

TIME: ____________

TOTAL CALORIES AT THIS MEAL:

TOTAL FAT AT THIS MEAL:

CARB:

VEGGIE:

PROTEIN:

BEVERAGE:

SNACK: ____________ TIME: ____________

LUNCH

TIME: ____________

TOTAL CALORIES AT THIS MEAL:

TOTAL FAT AT THIS MEAL:

CARB:

VEGGIE:

PROTEIN:

BEVERAGE:

SNACK: ____________ TIME: ____________

DINNER

TIME: ____________

TOTAL CALORIES AT THIS MEAL:

TOTAL FAT AT THIS MEAL:

CARB:

VEGGIE:

PROTEIN:

BEVERAGE:

SNACK: ____________ TIME: ____________

HOW DID I DO TODAY?

TOTAL STEPS:

STEP GOAL:

TOTAL CALORIES CONSUMED:

TOTAL CALORIES BURNED:

TOTAL FAT CONSUMED:

TOTAL FAT BURNED:

Daily Weight Loss Planner

Date: ______________   Calorie limit: ______ kcal | fat limit: ______ g

TO DO LIST:

TODAY'S WEIGHT:

TODAY'S WORKOUT WILL INCLUDE:

TYPE: DURATION:

☐ CARDIO: ______________ ______________

☐ RESISTANCE: ______________ ______________

☐ CLASS/OTHER ______________ ______________

BREAKFAST

TIME:

CARB:

VEGGIE:

PROTEIN:

BEVERAGE:

SNACK: TIME:

TOTAL CALORIES AT THIS MEAL:

TOTAL FAT AT THIS MEAL:

LUNCH

TIME:

CARB:

VEGGIE:

PROTEIN:

BEVERAGE:

SNACK: TIME:

TOTAL CALORIES AT THIS MEAL:

TOTAL FAT AT THIS MEAL:

DINNER

TIME:

CARB:

VEGGIE:

PROTEIN:

BEVERAGE:

SNACK: TIME:

TOTAL CALORIES AT THIS MEAL:

TOTAL FAT AT THIS MEAL:

HOW DID I DO TODAY?

TOTAL STEPS:

STEP GOAL:

TOTAL CALORIES CONSUMED:

TOTAL CALORIES BURNED:

TOTAL FAT CONSUMED:

TOTAL FAT BURNED:

Daily Weight Loss Planner

Date: Calorie limit: kcal | fat limit: g

TO DO LIST:

TODAY'S WORKOUT WILL INCLUDE:

TYPE: DURATION:

☐ **CARDIO:** _______________ _______________

☐ **RESISTANCE:** _______________ _______________

☐ **CLASS/OTHER** _______________ _______________

TODAY'S WEIGHT:

BREAKFAST

TIME: TOTAL CALORIES AT THIS MEAL: TOTAL FAT AT THIS MEAL:

CARB:

VEGGIE:

PROTEIN:

BEVERAGE:

SNACK: TIME:

LUNCH

TIME: TOTAL CALORIES AT THIS MEAL: TOTAL FAT AT THIS MEAL:

CARB:

VEGGIE:

PROTEIN:

BEVERAGE:

SNACK: TIME:

DINNER

TIME: TOTAL CALORIES AT THIS MEAL: TOTAL FAT AT THIS MEAL:

CARB:

VEGGIE:

PROTEIN:

BEVERAGE:

SNACK: TIME:

HOW DID I DO TODAY?

TOTAL STEPS: TOTAL CALORIES CONSUMED: TOTAL FAT CONSUMED:

STEP GOAL: TOTAL CALORIES BURNED: TOTAL FAT BURNED:

Daily Weight Loss Planner

Date:

Calorie limit: kcal | fat limit: g

TO DO LIST:

TODAY'S WEIGHT:

TODAY'S WORKOUT WILL INCLUDE:

TYPE: DURATION:

☐ CARDIO: _____________ _____________

☐ RESISTANCE: _____________ _____________

☐ CLASS/OTHER _____________ _____________

BREAKFAST

TIME:

CARB:

VEGGIE:

PROTEIN:

BEVERAGE:

SNACK: TIME:

TOTAL CALORIES AT THIS MEAL:

TOTAL FAT AT THIS MEAL:

LUNCH

TIME:

CARB:

VEGGIE:

PROTEIN:

BEVERAGE:

SNACK: TIME:

TOTAL CALORIES AT THIS MEAL:

TOTAL FAT AT THIS MEAL:

DINNER

TIME:

CARB:

VEGGIE:

PROTEIN:

BEVERAGE:

SNACK: TIME:

TOTAL CALORIES AT THIS MEAL:

TOTAL FAT AT THIS MEAL:

HOW DID I DO TODAY?

TOTAL STEPS:

STEP GOAL:

TOTAL CALORIES CONSUMED:

TOTAL CALORIES BURNED:

TOTAL FAT CONSUMED:

TOTAL FAT BURNED:

Daily Weight Loss Planner

Date: Calorie limit: kcal | fat limit: g

TO DO LIST:

TODAY'S WEIGHT:

TODAY'S WORKOUT WILL INCLUDE:

TYPE: DURATION:

☐ CARDIO: ____________ ____________

☐ RESISTANCE: ____________ ____________

☐ CLASS/OTHER ____________ ____________

BREAKFAST

TIME:

CARB:

VEGGIE:

PROTEIN:

BEVERAGE:

SNACK: TIME:

TOTAL CALORIES AT THIS MEAL:

TOTAL FAT AT THIS MEAL:

LUNCH

TIME:

CARB:

VEGGIE:

PROTEIN:

BEVERAGE:

SNACK: TIME:

TOTAL CALORIES AT THIS MEAL:

TOTAL FAT AT THIS MEAL:

DINNER

TIME:

CARB:

VEGGIE:

PROTEIN:

BEVERAGE:

SNACK: TIME:

TOTAL CALORIES AT THIS MEAL:

TOTAL FAT AT THIS MEAL:

HOW DID I DO TODAY?

TOTAL STEPS:

STEP GOAL:

TOTAL CALORIES CONSUMED:

TOTAL CALORIES BURNED:

TOTAL FAT CONSUMED:

TOTAL FAT BURNED:

Daily Weight Loss Planner

Date: Calorie limit: kcal | fat limit: g

TO DO LIST:

TODAY'S WORKOUT WILL INCLUDE:

TYPE: DURATION:

☐ CARDIO: ____________ ____________

☐ RESISTANCE: ____________ ____________

☐ CLASS/OTHER ____________ ____________

TODAY'S WEIGHT:

BREAKFAST

TIME:

CARB:

VEGGIE:

PROTEIN:

BEVERAGE:

SNACK: TIME:

TOTAL CALORIES AT THIS MEAL:

TOTAL FAT AT THIS MEAL:

LUNCH

TIME:

CARB:

VEGGIE:

PROTEIN:

BEVERAGE:

SNACK: TIME:

TOTAL CALORIES AT THIS MEAL:

TOTAL FAT AT THIS MEAL:

DINNER

TIME:

CARB:

VEGGIE:

PROTEIN:

BEVERAGE:

SNACK: TIME:

TOTAL CALORIES AT THIS MEAL:

TOTAL FAT AT THIS MEAL:

HOW DID I DO TODAY?

TOTAL STEPS:

STEP GOAL:

TOTAL CALORIES CONSUMED:

TOTAL CALORIES BURNED:

TOTAL FAT CONSUMED:

TOTAL FAT BURNED:

Daily Weight Loss Planner

Date: ___________   Calorie limit: ______ kcal | fat limit: ______ g

TO DO LIST:

TODAY'S WEIGHT:

TODAY'S WORKOUT WILL INCLUDE:

	TYPE:	DURATION:
☐ CARDIO:	___________	___________
☐ RESISTANCE:	___________	___________
☐ CLASS/OTHER	___________	___________

BREAKFAST

TIME: ___________

CARB:

VEGGIE:

PROTEIN:

BEVERAGE:

SNACK: ___________ TIME: ___________

TOTAL CALORIES AT THIS MEAL:

TOTAL FAT AT THIS MEAL:

LUNCH

TIME: ___________

CARB:

VEGGIE:

PROTEIN:

BEVERAGE:

SNACK: ___________ TIME: ___________

TOTAL CALORIES AT THIS MEAL:

TOTAL FAT AT THIS MEAL:

DINNER

TIME: ___________

CARB:

VEGGIE:

PROTEIN:

BEVERAGE:

SNACK: ___________ TIME: ___________

TOTAL CALORIES AT THIS MEAL:

TOTAL FAT AT THIS MEAL:

HOW DID I DO TODAY?

TOTAL STEPS:

STEP GOAL:

TOTAL CALORIES CONSUMED:

TOTAL CALORIES BURNED:

TOTAL FAT CONSUMED:

TOTAL FAT BURNED:

Daily Weight Loss Planner

Date: _______________

Calorie limit: _______ kcal | fat limit: _______ g

TO DO LIST:

TODAY'S WEIGHT:

TODAY'S WORKOUT WILL INCLUDE:

TYPE: | DURATION:

☐ CARDIO: _______________ _______________

☐ RESISTANCE: _______________ _______________

☐ CLASS/OTHER _______________ _______________

BREAKFAST
TIME:

CARB:

VEGGIE:

PROTEIN:

BEVERAGE:

SNACK: | TIME:

TOTAL CALORIES AT THIS MEAL:

TOTAL FAT AT THIS MEAL:

LUNCH
TIME:

CARB:

VEGGIE:

PROTEIN:

BEVERAGE:

SNACK: | TIME:

TOTAL CALORIES AT THIS MEAL:

TOTAL FAT AT THIS MEAL:

DINNER
TIME:

CARB:

VEGGIE:

PROTEIN:

BEVERAGE:

SNACK: | TIME:

TOTAL CALORIES AT THIS MEAL:

TOTAL FAT AT THIS MEAL:

HOW DID I DO TODAY?

TOTAL STEPS:

STEP GOAL:

TOTAL CALORIES CONSUMED:

TOTAL CALORIES BURNED:

TOTAL FAT CONSUMED:

TOTAL FAT BURNED:

Daily Weight Loss Planner

Date: | Calorie limit: ___ kcal | fat limit: ___ g

TO DO LIST:

TODAY'S WEIGHT:

TODAY'S WORKOUT WILL INCLUDE:

TYPE: | DURATION:

☐ CARDIO: ___________ ___________

☐ RESISTANCE: ___________ ___________

☐ CLASS/OTHER ___________ ___________

BREAKFAST

TIME:

CARB:

VEGGIE:

PROTEIN:

BEVERAGE:

SNACK: TIME:

TOTAL CALORIES AT THIS MEAL:

TOTAL FAT AT THIS MEAL:

LUNCH

TIME:

CARB:

VEGGIE:

PROTEIN:

BEVERAGE:

SNACK: TIME:

TOTAL CALORIES AT THIS MEAL:

TOTAL FAT AT THIS MEAL:

DINNER

TIME:

CARB:

VEGGIE:

PROTEIN:

BEVERAGE:

SNACK: TIME:

TOTAL CALORIES AT THIS MEAL:

TOTAL FAT AT THIS MEAL:

HOW DID I DO TODAY?

TOTAL STEPS:

STEP GOAL:

TOTAL CALORIES CONSUMED:

TOTAL CALORIES BURNED:

TOTAL FAT CONSUMED:

TOTAL FAT BURNED:

Daily Weight Loss Planner

Date:

Calorie limit: kcal | fat limit: g

TO DO LIST:

TODAY'S WEIGHT:

TODAY'S WORKOUT WILL INCLUDE:

TYPE: DURATION:

☐ CARDIO: ____________ ____________

☐ RESISTANCE: ____________ ____________

☐ CLASS/OTHER ____________ ____________

BREAKFAST

TIME:

CARB:

VEGGIE:

PROTEIN:

BEVERAGE:

SNACK: TIME:

TOTAL CALORIES AT THIS MEAL:

TOTAL FAT AT THIS MEAL:

LUNCH

TIME:

CARB:

VEGGIE:

PROTEIN:

BEVERAGE:

SNACK: TIME:

TOTAL CALORIES AT THIS MEAL:

TOTAL FAT AT THIS MEAL:

DINNER

TIME:

CARB:

VEGGIE:

PROTEIN:

BEVERAGE:

SNACK: TIME:

TOTAL CALORIES AT THIS MEAL:

TOTAL FAT AT THIS MEAL:

HOW DID I DO TODAY?

TOTAL STEPS:

STEP GOAL:

TOTAL CALORIES CONSUMED:

TOTAL CALORIES BURNED:

TOTAL FAT CONSUMED:

TOTAL FAT BURNED:

Notes:

Notes:

Notes:

About the Author

Rochelle Young, Registered/Licensed Dietitian; Owner/CEO of
Primary Nutrition Consulting LLC

To set up an individual nutrition consultation, contact by email:
primaryrdn@gmail.com

To order another copy of this planner and more, visit:
www.lulu.com

www.ingramcontent.com/pod-product-compliance
Lightning Source LLC
Chambersburg PA
CBHW081623250726
48657CB00009B/2696